LIVING THERAPY SERIES

Time Limited Therapy in Primary Care

A Person-Centred Dialogue

Richard Bryant-Jefferies

Radcliffe Medical Press

Radcliffe Medical Press Ltd
18 Marcham Road
Abingdon
Oxon OX14 1AA
United Kingdom

www.radcliffe-oxford.com
The Radcliffe Medical Press electronic catalogue and online ordering facility.
Direct sales to anywhere in the world.

British Library Cataloguing in Publication Data

A catalogue record for this book is available from the British Library.

ISBN 1 85775 999 0

Typeset by Aarontype Limited, Easton, Bristol
Printed and bound by TJ International Ltd, Padstow, Cornwall

Contents

Foreword

Many counsellors who work in primary care find it difficult to explain to colleagues in the primary healthcare team what they actually do with clients behind the closed door of their room. It's so easy for these other team members – nurses, doctors, health visitors, receptionists and managers. Their work is understood for the most part by both the recipients of care and by each team member who knows what others do. The outcomes of their activities can be measured and for the most part each professional understands and respects the work of the others as they more often than not share common aims and objectives in delivering healthcare.

For the counsellor, the task of explaining is much more difficult. How can you explain what empathy, congruence and unconditional positive regard bring to the relationship between counsellor and client in a healthcare environment, where so often therapeutic success is measured by adherence to treatment guidelines, protocols and easy-to-measure outcomes? What are the outcomes of counselling and why should the service be in primary healthcare? What is measured by other members of the primary healthcare team usually has a physical presence, dependent on diagnosis reached by an informed interpretation of symptoms and physical signs, and validated or confirmed by investigations, blood tests, scans and X-rays.

Unfortunately, the patients usually referred to counsellors by GPs have a range of symptoms which have no such physical signs, and their symptoms can be interpreted in many ways by the referrer, dependent on his or her experience, prejudice and even the feelings evoked in the mind of the referrer by the patient. The labelling used – 'heartsink patients', the 'worried well', 'personality disorder', 'frequent attender' – are good examples of this tendency.

In this book the author brings to life in a gripping way what really does go on when a counsellor sees a patient in the primary healthcare setting, where, usually, arbitrary, externally defined constraints on session length and on the number of sessions offered are in place and expectations are that somehow the patient will be fixed or even cured.

The text consists of an imaginary dialogue between a patient and therapist, as well as the dialogue between the counsellor and supervisor, illustrating the parallel process. For me, what was so surprising was my engagement in yet another level of parallel process as I read the unfolding story. It's not a description of a brilliant therapist doing things to a grateful client who gains wonderful insights that change her life. Instead, it tells the story of a therapeutic relationship as it often is.

The therapist makes mistakes, the client fails to keep appointments and the therapist is often puzzled by what goes on, but the shared endeavour in the end, with the help of some excellent supervision, produces a satisfactory conclusion.

The model of therapy described is person-centred and, as you would expect, stresses congruence, empathy and unconditional regard. As a description of a therapeutic relationship that had a beneficial outcome it cannot be faulted. Yet, of course, these common factors are or should be present whatever the therapy modality used whenever effective counselling takes place (needing only the addition of what Scott Miller and his colleagues call the 'heroic client' to produce a desirable outcome, as was the case in the book).

For once it's good to read a book that describes so realistically and movingly the minute-by-minute account of what actually happened, not a book describing clever therapists getting it right all the time. As the story unfolds the common humanity of both client and therapist shines through, which is a measure of the author's success, bringing to life so convincingly the imaginary encounter. Maybe the book should be required reading for newly appointed non-clinical managers of counselling services (which is unfortunately becoming increasingly common), and for primary healthcare staff about to start working with a counsellor as a member of their team. Students too would find a lot to think about, and the questions at the end of each section are a useful tool for self-learning and reflection.

Graham Curtis Jenkins
Director
Counselling in Primary Care Trust
General Practitioner (retired)
May 2003

Foreword

Richard Bryant-Jefferies has undertaken a difficult task with this book. It is an effort that sets out to delineate the foundations and clinical work of person-centered counsellors in a practice setting. This inauspicious task is even more demanding in that Bryant-Jefferies' main thrust is to identify the person-centered approach in relation to time limited therapy. Within this task, he delineates client problem and process and, as well, therapist function and process.

His work represents an in-depth knowledge about, and experience with, operating as a person-centered therapist (counsellor) in a real and practical setting. He takes the reader through the client–therapist process as experienced in the 'real' world. He offers the therapist's inner struggles including exploration of the therapist's feelings and thoughts with a person-centered supervisor.

Richard presents the organizational setting as a context that accepts, but is overall not especially congruent with, the operational base and assumptions of the person-centered approach. It is a notable observation that a medically oriented and directive organization can become receptive to the work of the person-centered counsellor. In addition, he offers large remnants of the way that sessions might go with a particular client by providing client–therapist dialogue and periodic comments about the six sessions. He includes some of the thoughts and feelings of both therapist and client. The six sessions are the maximum number of sessions typically available to clients in this setting. Thus, the counsellor is forced to deal with 'time limited therapy'. There is a subtle display of Richard's frustration with the limited sessions generally accorded to the clients, but there is also satisfaction that the person-centered approach restricted by time limited conditions is clinically effective.

Bryant-Jefferies suggests that it may be difficult to capture the real depth and experience from some of the verbal interactions and counsellor's comments. I think that this is a point especially true of any particular client-centered therapy session wherein the most boring session from an outsider's view is often the most meaningful to the client. Perhaps, as a way to counter this outsider view, Richard periodically expresses a bias towards feelings, specific process and emotionally charged content. Some 'pure' person-centered/client-centered therapists are likely to question this periodic emphasis from the fundamental non-directive theory of Rogers (1959). Some of the emphases of the counsellor and, especially, much of the directionality of the person-centered supervisor as characterized in the supervisory discourse digress from the fundamental axiom of Rogers' theory, albeit congruent to some of the viable tributaries of the theory. Presentation of the type offered in this book might confuse the person-centered therapist's 'doing' with 'being'. This is always a difficulty when one attempts to explain the person-centered approach. It behooves us to remember that the theory of client-centered therapy is predicated upon the therapeutic axiom of certain therapist attitudes; that is, the congruent therapist's *experiencing* of unconditional positive regard towards the client and empathic understanding of the client's frame of reference (1959). This is the *sine qua non* of the person-centered approach. It is not the particular empathic responses that necessarily convey the therapist's experiences of the client. It is not the directionality to develop any particular direction to the client's way, pace or direction. Richard acknowledges this several times in his practice delineation. Attitudes are difficult to demonstrate with verbal summations, and particularly difficult to communicate to the general problem-oriented, medically determined treatment of professionals. Given these portentous barriers, Bryant-Jefferies has soundly accomplished a difficult undertaking.

Jerold D Bozarth PhD
Professor Emeritus
University of Georgia
USA
May 2003

Preface

Recent years have seen an increase in the use of what has become termed 'time limited' therapy, particularly, although not exclusively, in primary healthcare settings. Many employee assistance programmes (EAPs) also employ a time limited method of working. However, not all counsellors will have experienced this way of working either in their training or their practice.

This book provides the reader with an insight into the process of counselling and the issues that can arise when working in a time limited way. It is set within a primary healthcare setting, and presents the reader with not just insight, but hopefully experience of the process of counselling and the factors that need to be taken into account when working as a counsellor within this environment.

As well as offering material that will be helpful in training, this book also offers genuine insight for experienced counsellors and other healthcare professionals working alongside counsellors, particularly in GP surgeries. The book includes fictitious dialogue between a client and her counsellor, and the counsellor and his supervisor, examples of notes from each counselling session, a series of points for discussion and boxed comments highlighting significant factors or experiences that emerge during the process, and how they might be responded to. Like other books in the *Living Therapy* series, *Time Limited Therapy in Primary Care: a person-centred dialogue* will contribute to demystifying the therapy, and at the same time provides useful approaches and frameworks that may be used by professionals other than counsellors.

The person-centred theoretical model provides the basis for the counselling work described, and a brief overview of this is given in the introduction. This approach has been chosen simply because it is my own core model and one that offers attitudinal values at its heart, which I believe to be crucial in helping people, and which research has clearly indicated to be an effective way of working.

As well as being useful for professionals, this book will also help clients, or potential clients, to inform themselves about what they might expect from person-centred counselling within this professional context and within a time limited framework.

Richard Bryant-Jefferies
May 2003

About the author

Richard Bryant-Jefferies qualified in person-centred counselling in 1994 and remains passionate about the application and effectiveness of this approach. He has been working in a GP surgery as a general counsellor for a number of years and has an appreciation first hand of the challenges and opportunities of establishing such a service in a GP surgery, and of the value it can have.

Richard also has experience of working with clients with alcohol problems (in primary healthcare settings) and as well as counselling within this specialism, he also supervises counsellors who work with people with drug and alcohol problems, and has a general counselling supervision practice. He offers 'Alcohol Awareness and Response' workshops nationally for both counsellors and other professionals.

Richard has had articles published in journals including *BACP*, *HCPJ*, *Practice Nurse*, and had his first book on a counselling theme published in 2001, *Counselling the Person Beyond the Alcohol Problem* (Jessica Kingsley Publishers), providing theoretical yet practical insights into the application of the person-centred approach within the context of the 'cycle of change' model that has been widely adopted to describe the process of change.

Since then he has been writing for the *Living Therapy* series, the first book in this series being *Problem Drinking: a person-centred dialogue* followed by *Counselling a Survivor of Child Sexual Abuse* and *Counselling a Recovering Drug User*. This series of books aims to bring therapy alive, to transport the reader into the counselling sessions and to gain an experience of engaging with the characters and the process, as a result gaining greater awareness of themselves through their own reactions and responses.

Richard is keen to bring the experience of the therapeutic process, from the perspective of this approach, to a wider audience. He is concerned to demonstrate its application in various settings and to address a range of specific issues. Richard is convinced that the attitudinal values of the person-centred approach and the emphasis it places on the *therapeutic relationship* which offers opportunity for greater self-awareness and reduced incongruence, are key to helping people resolve difficulties.

Therapy is a process. We do not know where it will lead. But if we offer the person who is our client a supportive and accepting climate of relationship, if we are authentic with them and can convey empathic understanding of their inner and outer world, then the possibility of movement towards a more complete sense of self and a more satisfying experience in life becomes possible.

Acknowledgements

I wish to thank June Richards for reading through my first draft and offering insightful comments, which were gratefully received. My thanks also to John Eatock for casting his eye over the introduction and making helpful suggestions.

Disclaimer

The characters in this book (Mandy, Martin and Anne) are fictitious and are not intended to bear resemblance to any particular person or persons.

Introduction

This title, the second in the *Living Therapy* series, again utilises fictitious dialogue between a counsellor and his client, and the counsellor and his supervisor, to describe the person-centred counselling process as it might occur within a six-session time limited framework. The setting is a GP surgery. The aim is to enable the reader not only to gain insight into this process, but also to engage at an emotional level with what is occurring within each person and the therapeutic relationships that are present.

The theoretical model for time limited therapy presented in this book is that of the person-centred approach (PCA) founded by Carl Rogers. The approach is widely used by counsellors working in the UK today: in a membership survey conducted by the British Association for Counselling and Psychotherapy in 2001, 35.6 per cent of those responding claimed to work to the PCA, while 25.4 per cent identified themselves as psychodynamic practitioners. The approach might be described as a non-directive, relational approach to counselling, unique in many ways among counselling models as it does not set the therapist up as an expert or work towards a specific goal. Rather the aim of the person-centred counsellor is to offer a facilitative environment such that the client's own developmental potential can be released to find its own fulfilling expression. The theory underlying the PCA is described later in this introduction.

The client, Mandy, recently broke down in tears when seeing her GP. The problem that she presented to her GP was concerned with work stress, and the GP decided to refer her to Martin, the surgery counsellor. The client has experienced significant losses in her life, and while these were not the primary motivation for the referral, they become relevant factors within the therapeutic journey. As is often the case in primary healthcare referrals for counselling, the presenting issues can be the tip of a difficult iceberg, and it is only as the client begins to talk about their feelings that other relevant experiences come to the surface. This, in itself, can present a huge challenge to time limited working, as what may on the surface appear to require six sessions of counselling turns out to involve deep-seated emotional traumas that may take much longer to resolve. The issues that arise from this are dealt with later.

Martin is a person-centred counsellor. He has worked in this GP surgery for a number of years and has a good working relationship with all the GPs. He has fortnightly supervision sessions with Anne, his supervisor. In counselling, regular ongoing supervision is a professional requirement. It provides an opportunity for counsellors to process and explore emotional reactions to their work, reflect on their practice in terms of their core theory, seek a fellow professional's perspective on dilemmas that arise, and gain general support as a human being in working with often painful and traumatic experiences presented by their clients.

Anne has herself worked in GP surgeries and appreciates some of the difficulties and challenges that the environment presents. She, like Martin, works to the theory and attitudinal qualities of the PCA. She has worked with Martin for three years and has grown to appreciate his style of working and his integrity as a counsellor.

The supervision sessions are included because they are an integral part of the therapeutic process. It is also hoped that they will help readers from other professions to recognise the value of some form of supportive and collaborative supervision and thus help them to become more authentically present with their own clients.

Readers who are unfamiliar with counselling may at first find it unusual that many of Martin's responses to Mandy seem to be simple reflections of what she has said. Martin is voicing empathic responses, often with a sense of 'checking out' that he is hearing accurately what the client is saying. The client says something; the counsellor then conveys what he has heard, sometimes with the same words, sometimes including a sense of what he feels may be being communicated through the client's tone of voice, facial expression or simply the atmosphere of the moment. The client is then enabled to confirm that they have been heard accurately, or to correct the counsellor in his perception. The client may then explore more deeply what they have been saying or move on, in either case with a sense that they have been heard and warmly accepted.

The person-centred approach

The PCA was formulated by Carl Rogers. He proposed that certain conditions, when present within a therapeutic relationship, would enable the client to develop towards what he termed 'fuller functionality'. Over a number of years he refined these ideas, which he defined as 'the necessary and sufficient conditions for constructive personality change'. He described these conditions in a paper in the late 1950s. They are:

1 Two persons are in psychological contact.
2 The first, whom we shall term the client, is in a state of incongruence, being vulnerable or anxious.
3 The second person, whom we shall term the therapist, is congruent or integrated in the relationship.
4 The therapist experiences unconditional positive regard for the client.
5 The therapist experiences an empathic understanding of the client's internal frame of reference and endeavours to communicate this experience to the client.

6   The communication to the client of the therapist's empathic understanding
and unconditional positive regard is to a minimal degree achieved (Rogers,
1957, p.96).

Rogers defined empathy as meaning 'entering the private perceptual world of
the other ... being sensitive, moment by moment, to the changing felt meanings
which flow in this other person. ... It means sensing meanings of which he or she
is scarcely aware, but not trying to uncover totally unconscious feelings' (Rogers,
1980, p.142). It is a very delicate process, and it provides, I believe, a foundation
block. The counsellor's role is primarily to establish empathic rapport and communicate empathic understanding to the client.

Within this relationship the counsellor seeks to maintain an attitude of unconditional positive regard towards the client whatever they disclose. This is not
'agreeing with', it is the offering of a sincere and warm acceptance. Rogers wrote,
'when the therapist is experiencing a positive, acceptant attitude towards whatever the client *is* at that moment, therapeutic movement or change is more likely
to occur' (Rogers, 1980, p.116). Mearns and Thorne suggest that 'unconditional
positive regard is the label given to the fundamental attitude of the person-
centred counsellor towards her client. The counsellor who holds this attitude
deeply values the humanity of her client and is not deflected in that valuing by
any particular client behaviours. The attitude manifests itself in the counsellor's
consistent acceptance of and enduring warmth towards her client' (Mearns and
Thorne, 1988, p.59).

Last, but by no means least, is that state of being that Rogers referred to as congruence, but which has also been described in terms of 'realness', 'transparency',
'genuineness', and 'authenticity'. Indeed, Rogers wrote that '... genuineness,
realness or congruence ... this means that the therapist is openly being the feelings and attitudes that are flowing within at the moment ... the term transparent
catches the flavour of this condition.' Putting this into the therapeutic setting, we
can say that 'congruence is the state of being of the counsellor when her outward
responses to her client consistently match the inner feelings and sensations
which she has in relation to her client' (Mearns and Thorne, 1999).

I would suggest that any congruent expression by the counsellor of their feelings or reactions has to emerge through the process of being in therapeutic relationship with the client. It is a disciplined response and not an open door to
endless self-disclosure. Congruent expression is perhaps most appropriate and
therapeutically valuable where it is informed by the existence of an empathic
understanding of the client's inner world, and is offered in a climate of a genuinely
warm acceptance towards the client. In other words, that which becomes present
within the counsellor, and is transparently offered to the client, emerges through
the counsellor's empathic sensitivity to the client's inner frame of reference.

PCA regards the relationship that we have with our clients, and the attitude
that we hold within that relationship, to be key factors. In my experience, many
problems develop out of life experiences that involve problematic relational
experiences. This can be centred in childhood or later in life. What is important
is that the individual, through relationships that have a negative conditioning

effect, is left with a distorted perception of themselves and their potential as a person. I see many people who, from their childhood experiences, have learned beliefs such as 'I can never be good enough to be praised for what I have achieved; I never match my parents' expectations', or 'No one was ever there for me when I was hurting; perhaps I am unlovable'. The result is a loss of a positive sense of self, and the individual adapts to maintain the newly learned concept of self. This is then lived out, possibly throughout life, the person seeking to satisfy what they have come to believe about themselves: being unable to achieve, feeling unable to be loved, though perhaps in both cases maintaining a constant desperation to receive what they never had. Yet, perversely, they may then sabotage any possibility of gaining what they want in order to maintain the negatively conditioned sense of self.

It is my belief that by offering someone a non-judgemental, warm, accepting and authentic relationship, the person can grow into a fresh sense of self in which their potential as a person can become more fulfilled. Such an experience fosters an opportunity for the client to redefine themselves as they experience the presence of the therapist's congruence, empathy and unconditional positive regard. This process can take time. Often the personality change that is required to sustain a shift away from what have been termed 'conditions of worth' requires a lengthy period of therapeutic work, bearing in mind that the person may be struggling to unravel a sense of self that has been developed, sustained and reinforced for many decades of life. This presents a challenge to time limited working. However, where the length of time is clear, it is my belief that the client can be trusted to adjust to that time frame and to use it for their benefit.

The term 'conditions of worth' applies to the conditioning that is frequently present in childhood, and at other times in life, when a person experiences that their worth is conditional on doing something, or behaving, in a certain way. This is usually to satisfy someone else's needs, and can be contrary to the client's own sense of what would be a satisfying experience. The values of others become a feature of the individual's structure of self. It can have the effect of generating anxiety as the person moves away from being true to themselves, learning instead to remain 'true' to their conditioned sense of worth.

Is the person-centred approach to counselling and psychotherapy effective? During the 1950s and 1960s Rogers and his associates devised methodologies and designed measuring instruments with the specific intent of investigating psychotherapy. A recent review of research into client-centred psychotherapy (Bozarth et al., 2002, p. 179) concluded that 'research has supported the theory that a congruent therapist's experience of empathic understanding of the client's frame of reference and experience of unconditional positive regard are related to positive outcome'. In terms of primary care settings, 'Rowland et al. (2000) in the vital Cochrane review, established the effectiveness of counselling in primary care settings for the treatment of patients with depression. This review used studies in which person-centred counselling was the major approach' (BAPCA, 2000).

A randomised controlled trial was also conducted in 2000 to compare person-centred counselling, cognitive behavioural therapy and routine general practitioner care (King et al., 2000). The subject group were patients suffering from depression, and mixed anxiety and depression. Their findings, as reported in BAPCA (2000), were that 'there was no difference in therapeutic effectiveness' between the two therapies, that at the four-month follow-up both obtained 'significantly better results than "usual general practitioner care"', 'higher patient satisfaction scores were recorded for the psychological therapies', 'there was no difference in the cost-effectiveness in the three treatments although Professor King concluded "... the significantly greater clinical effectiveness of the psychological therapies at four months means that these [psychological] treatments are more cost-effective methods of reducing depressive symptoms in the short term [than usual GP care]"'.

While I would be interested in reading the results of longer-term studies to ascertain which theoretical approaches have longer-lasting effects, I am also mindful that depression and anxiety are often reactions to circumstances, and the resolving of these symptoms at one point in life may not necessarily mean that a person will not experience the symptoms again in relation to other circumstances (or the same ones) at a later date. My instinct is that approaches that include the resolution of underlying issues as well as changing cognition and behaviour in the present are more likely to have a longer-lasting effect.

I am also aware of the difficulty in researching an approach to counselling that is centred very much on *the experience of the client in relationship with a particular therapist*. Randomised controlled trials can struggle to cater for the subjective, relational variable that emerges when two people encounter each other in the counselling room. What occurs is a unique experience. Comparison with other unique encounters can take us so far, but what needs to be grasped are those experiential factors that contributed to constructive personality change. It is a fact that human beings find themselves more in tune with some people than others, and this is as true in the therapy room as anywhere else.

The PCA, it seems to me, lends itself to qualitative research based on case studies and the experience of individual clients. The client is surely best placed to be able to report what, for them, was experienced as the most significant feature of a counselling encounter with a person-centred therapist. I would argue that person-centred counselling is at least as much an art as a science, and perhaps more so. The subjective perceptions of the client as they enter into relationship with a therapist will hold the key to greater understanding of what has been helpful. Effectiveness of the counselling relationship may be more about how the therapist *is* rather than what he or she *does*. And in comparing and contrasting different approaches, effective therapy may be less about the nature of a given therapy and more about the very personhood of the therapist themselves. It is also important to remember that the very philosophy of the PCA means that the counsellor is working, as the name suggests, with a 'person-centred' rather than a 'problem-centred' focus.

This is obviously a very brief introduction to the approach. Person-centred theory continues to develop as practitioners and theoreticians consider its application in various fields of therapeutic work. Much has been, and continues to be, written about the PCA and a reading list of suggested titles is included at the end of this book.

Assessment and diagnosis

The first session in this dialogue does not include a lengthy assessment. The counsellor seeks to work towards building the therapeutic relationship by allowing the client to communicate what is pressing for her. Untimely assessment can cut across a person-centred way of working which is rooted in a trust that the client will bring to sessions what material he or she feels a need and a readiness to address. It is also a fact that this approach is more concerned with building a therapeutic relationship with the person and allowing the presence of the therapeutic conditions to effect constructive personality change, than with the counsellor 'doing' something specific to alleviate a given set of symptoms or focusing solely on a specific problem.

In my experience, lengthy assessments that involve a whole battery of questions can get in the way of building the therapeutic relationship and allowing the client to 'tell their story'. Generally, I find that much of the information relevant to the client's difficulties is communicated as the session proceeds. In contrast, the often 'question-and-answer' tone of assessment can set a pattern for the counselling relationship and can have the effect of forcing disclosures from clients before they are ready, or feel trusting of the therapist, to share this information. The power balance is therefore very much biased towards the counsellor. The PCA, on the other hand, seeks to equalise the power balance, for this is a key element of the therapeutic relationship.

Others will take the view that without a full assessment the counsellor will not know whether the client requires a counselling response that may be outside that counsellor's sphere of competence or how much that client is a risk to themselves or to others. Casemore (2002) refers to an earlier article (Casemore, 2000) and argues that counsellors should not begin counselling unless they are clear that they can reach 'an acceptable point of closure' within the time frame given, and that there should be a more 'rigorous assessment and diagnosis to determine whether realistic outcomes can be achieved within six to eight weeks'. He goes on to suggest that where this is not the case, that to begin counselling 'would be unethical'.

There remains a debate also as to whether diagnosis can necessarily be trusted and empirical when it comes to mental health factors. Bozarth (2002) refers to his own studies of particular diagnostic concepts which do not evidence the clustering of symptoms in a meaningful way (Bozarth, 1998) and to those of others in relation to schizophrenia (Bentall, 1990; Slade and Cooper, 1979), depression (Hallett, 1990; Wiener, 1989), agoraphobia (Hallam, 1983), borderline personality disorder (Kutchins and Kirk, 1997) and panic disorder (Hallam, 1989).

What may be a panic disorder today that seems connected to a traumatic incident the previous week may still have its roots in far deeper trauma from earlier in life, trauma which the client may not currently be ready to address, or even remember. From the person-centred perspective I would argue that clients know what they need to deal with, what is causing them disturbance in the present. They may not feel ready to address other deep-seated issues at this time, but they may become ready to do so in the future, at a time that is right for their own process of being. The very experience of counselling may enable the client to feel able to voice that which they had previously kept hidden, or which had kept itself hidden.

So clients may attend for counselling without full awareness of the scope of their difficulty, or the nature of underlying factors that may only come to light through the process of therapy. What they do not disclose may either be because they do not feel able to address this within a time limited framework or they may simply be unaware of some experience that has become dissociated. While it may provoke symptoms of discomfort, it is not at this time producing the degree of pain or dysfunction that may force them to address it. I have also heard it said by colleagues that allowing clients time and space to tell their own story in their own way and at their own pace tends to allow all that might have been revealed through a specific assessment to be brought into the open anyway. Sometimes the whole therapy can be the very process of the client 'telling their story' and feeling heard, understood and warmly accepted by another person.

Counsellors need to be sensitive to the psychological processes that are present within the client. Very often it is the timing of good therapy that is important. The client may well have to be emotionally, mentally, psychologically and even spiritually in the right frame of reference within themselves in order to engage in productive counselling. This frame of reference, from a person-centred perspective, would involve the presence of a state of incongruence within the client producing symptoms ranging through depression, anxiety, stress, panic and the so-called 'borderline personality disorder'. This latter seems, at times, to have become the catch-all for those whose behaviour does not fit a diagnosis, yet which seems diffi-cult to treat by conventional means. Many of the people I have worked with who carry this diagnostic label have experienced severe trauma of a physical and/or emotional nature, and have, in seeking to alleviate their symptoms, frequently exacerbated them through the use of drugs and/or alcohol.

In some services, the client will have already been assessed by another team member prior to counselling. This often happens in employee assistance pro-grammes (EAPs) and can occur within NHS psychological therapy departments, the latter generally being multidisciplinary and including psychologists (some with specialisms), psychotherapists and counsellors. The counsellor is then being given only relevant information, although an assessment has taken place to try to ascertain suitability for counselling and, in the context of this book, time limited counselling. The counsellor makes this information visible to the client. Transparency can then be maintained and the therapeutic relationship can be built at the client's pace with the client deciding on the content of sessions. Nevertheless, issues will still arise that the client may feel are pressing and want to discuss, which are essentially the tip of a volcano waiting to erupt beyond the boundary of time limited working.

The truth is, surely, that assessment is an ongoing process; clients change over time and the counsellor needs to be vigilant to this. This ongoing perspective of continuous assessment throughout the counselling process where the client is involved can have therapeutic value. In an article published in *Counselling in Practice*, Scott D Miller and colleagues described their work in bringing the clients' experiences of therapy more fully into the foreground of clinical practice. They write, 'We involved our clients in a session-by-session evaluation of both their satisfaction with and progress in treatment. With rare exceptions, our clients were willing and interested participants. As one man said, "Hey, we're evaluating you anyway!" The difference, however, was that assessment no longer preceded and dictated the intervention but became an on-going, collaborative process as pivotal to treatment as change itself' (Miller *et al.*, 2001).

Rogers also questioned the value of psychological diagnosis. He argued that it could place the client's locus of value firmly outside themselves and definitely within the diagnosing 'expert', leaving the client at risk of developing tendencies of dependence and expectation that the 'expert' will have the responsibility of improving the client's situation (Rogers, 1951, p.223). He also formulated the following propositional statements:

> Behaviour is caused, and the psychological cause of behaviour is a certain perception or a way of perceiving.
> The client is the only one who has the potentiality of knowing fully the dynamics of his perceptions and his behaviour.
> In order for behaviour to change, a change in perception must be *experienced*. Intellectual knowledge cannot substitute for this.
> The constructive forces which bring about altered perception, reorganization of self, and relearning, reside primarily in the client, and probably cannot come from outside.
> Therapy is basically the experiencing of the inadequacies in old ways of perceiving, the experiencing of new and more accurate and adequate perceptions, and the recognition of significant relationship between perceptions.
> In a very meaningful and accurate sense, therapy *is* diagnosis, and this diagnosis is a process which goes on in the experience of the client, rather than in the intellect of the clinician. (Rogers, 1951, pp.221–3)

Time limited counselling

What does this term actually mean? How does 'time limited' contrast with 'brief' or 'short-term' therapy? As the name implies, it is counselling that is offered within a given time frame, the length of time being the limiting factor. It is not necessarily what has become termed 'brief therapy', which is a specific technique for working with clients over a short period of time. Time limited therapy can involve the application of a wide range of therapeutic models; they are simply being offered within a specific and limited period of time. Short-term counselling might be viewed as having another meaning again. Here we do not have anything suggestive of limitation. It may therefore be regarded as having greater flexibility.

In a published letter, Mearns (2002) refers to the experience of the Lanarkshire Counselling Service, a primary care counselling service in 54 general practices.

He suggests that 'it is perfectly possible to run a primary care counselling service on a short-term basis without it being time-limited'. He defines short-term counselling as a service that works to, for instance, an average client contact time of six hours, distinguishing this from a time limited approach which would adhere to a rigid six hours maximum per client.

Clearly, short-term working provides far greater flexibility for the counsellor and the client, and with this comes the possibility, when deep-seated issues arise, of spending more time working at greater depth on those issues or, where it is deemed necessary, having an appropriate length of time to seek and prepare for a longer therapeutic process elsewhere and provide a realistic time frame for closure. Issues of deep significance can arise in the final session of six, and short-term working can offer the flexible response of time for the client to consider their options in an ethical and therapeutic way.

My own experience of working within GP surgeries is that I have tended more towards 'short-term' working. Generally speaking, what I offer is an initial contract for a maximum of six sessions, and around the fourth session this will be reviewed to ascertain whether further counselling is likely to be helpful. Some clients wish for more, others do not. Fortunately, I have flexibility that enables me to work well beyond the six sessions in cases where I, the client and the referring GP feel this will be therapeutically valuable.

I would not wish to work to a rigid six-session time frame for all clients referred to me, although I recognise that this can be helpful, and have worked with many people within this agreed time frame. However, I am grateful for the flexibility, should it be required, if a related (or unrelated) issue arises that is relevant to the client's mental and emotional health, and which is within my sphere of competence.

As well as wishing to provide readers with an experience of working within a time limited framework in a primary healthcare setting, one of the main motivating factors in writing this book has been to highlight the tensions that can arise and the issues that need to be considered when offering a counselling service in this way. My belief is that time limited work can be helpful, but it should not become a universal panacea for effective counselling. I favour the short-term counselling model as argued for by Mearns (2002), and hope that while this book demonstrates practice within a time limited framework, it nevertheless leaves the reader with a sense that perhaps greater flexibility could have offered more to the client. I will return to this in the conclusion.

Why has time limited working become a feature of counselling, not only in primary healthcare but also in other areas, such as within EAPs? The truth is that the major factor is cost. As an ex-fundholding manager I am well aware of the debates taking place over what service to buy to help patients with mental and emotional health problems. In fundholding, money needed to be vired from mental health budgets into counselling services, and there was a limit to what could be offered. In many respects, six sessions was seen as better than nothing, a step in the direction of greater therapeutic emphasis in treatment responses. The advantage of a counsellor within the GP surgery made the service more accessible to people, and made it easier for people to accept referral without the stigma of seeing a professional from a 'mental health service'. I still see people who remain concerned that referral to a mental health team would appear on their notes and remain a problematic factor when health reports are required, for instance for employment or insurance purposes.

Today we are seeing the establishment of National Service Frameworks and the increasing emphasis on clinical governance, regulation and other guidance from government. Standards are being sought. Indeed, standards are required, and patients should be able to know that the counselling they receive is from practitioners who are effective in their field, and who work in ways that are demonstrably effective. Richardson (2001) sets out the governmental agenda, highlighting the importance of public protection and professional standards, along with the need for clear consensus, agreement on registration criteria and mechanisms for registration. There is also emphasis on the role of professional self-regulation. Yet there are also voices of concern about regulation. Thorne (2002a, p.5) argues passionately that 'regulation in the hands of government or the law would inevitably mean a stifling of creativity and the proliferation of therapists who can no longer offer the best of themselves for fear of making mistakes or earning adverse judgement in an increasingly litigious society'.

Distinctions are being drawn between which patients with which problems should be referred for counselling and which for psychiatric intervention. There is a belief that specific conditions respond to specific therapeutic treatments. The time offered for counselling has become a feature of this. Yet it has been argued strongly that within the mental health context specific treatments for specific dysfunctions are a myth (Bozarth, 2002). In his conclusion, Bozarth calls for a 'radical restructuring of the mental health system [USA] to accentuate the variables related to success. These are the common factor variables of therapist/client relationship and emphasis of client resources and the client's frame of reference.' If we begin to accept that not all 'diagnoses' are necessarily robust but actually much more subjectively based, then we create the opportunity to change an important mindset, namely we can begin to think more in terms of the 'person' as a whole rather than simply a 'medical diagnostic label'.

In person-centred working the emphasis is placed on process and the centrality of the client's experiencing and perception. Each client will have their own unique set of experiences and meanings that they have developed through life experience. With increasing emphasis placed on 'evidence-based practice' perhaps we should also emphasise 'practice-based evidence', with increasing focus on qualitative research, recognising the uniqueness of each individual client and counsellor, and the encounter between them in therapy.

How do GPs view time limited counselling? My experience of working alongside GPs makes it clear to me that what the GP wants more than anything else is a treatment response that is helpful to his or her patients. I have heard it said how much they value the presence of a counsellor within the surgery. As one GP wrote, 'The counselling service has demonstrated to us, over the last two years, the effective contribution that can be made by a counsellor to a primary care team. In acknowledging this work we are aware of the extensive hours it has saved us, of the comfort of having quick access to a counsellor and of the appreciation expressed by patients for this service.' A GP's fundamental concern is the health of their patients. Yet GPs also want to be sure that what is being offered is not only effective from the standpoint of health, but also from the standpoint of cost.

Curtis Jenkins (2002) provides an extremely helpful overview of the difficulties related to developing, applying and interpreting research trials into the effectiveness of counselling. It is an area fraught with problems, including difficulties in achieving genuine randomisation, researcher bias, too small sample sizes, publication bias, difficulties associated with the interpretation of data and outcomes, and standardisation of the types of therapy interventions. He comments, with reference to Asay and Lambert (1999), that 'the reality is that most psychotherapy researchers now reluctantly agree that therapists themselves are more likely to be the cause of outcome variance than the style or type of therapy offered'.

It seems to me that the positive effects of time limited therapy are likely to be more than simply those related directly to the presenting symptoms. There is a process of learning and of emotional maturation that can extend into other areas of a person's inner and outer world that can have a cost-effectiveness beyond just health factors. This could include improved work performance, greater effectiveness as a parent and reduction in problematic behaviours that are a cost to society.

If, during the time limited period, it emerges that the client has issues that may need to be dealt with by longer-term counselling, this should be discussed. The client may decide that they do not wish to engage with these other areas, preferring to work within the six-session framework with the original focus. Others may agree to additional counselling, and in this case the remaining sessions can usefully be utilised to prepare the client for that longer period of counselling or other therapy.

Referral is made back to the GP to consider options: agreement for further sessions or referral on to a specialist service, where appropriate. The client may be given the option of private counselling where there is no NHS provision available. In their BACP information sheet, Palmer and Mander indicate that the 'ethical way to handle this is to provide them with an independent list of counsellors and services'. It is important that the client is free to make their own choice. The information sheet stresses that 'no pressure should be put on them to continue with the current counsellor in a private capacity'. Ideally, the transition will be smooth. However, access to a longer period of counselling or psychotherapy may require the client to go on a waiting list. Where this is the case, it can be useful to use the remaining sessions to establish what the client needs to help them cope with the time gap in service provision.

The risk in this situation is that the client is left with unresolved issues, or perhaps an experience of being hurried through the process (either by themselves, or maybe by a counsellor affected by the constraint of the time frame). I can, however, imagine how a rigid six-session limit will exacerbate tension within the counsellor (and the client) to achieve a successful outcome.

I rather feel that sometimes what the counsellor, the health service and the client would define as being 'a success' differs. In this book, the client may feel that getting back to work is their success, for the GP it may be the eradication of the anxiety symptoms, for the counsellor it could be the sense that the client has achieved a fuller measure of congruence, for the health service the National Institute of Clinical Excellence (NICE) may be more concerned with whether the health outcome is cost-effective in terms of 'health costs'.

For the person-centred counsellor, the process of counselling will be client led, with, as highlighted earlier, trust in the client to know what their needs are and what they wish to address within the remaining sessions. This is important, and a crucial feature of the approach. Taking the theoretical position that each person has within them, or is subject to, an 'actualising process' or, as Rogers tempered it, an 'actualising tendency', a tendency towards fuller and more complete personhood with an associated greater fulfilment of their potentialities, we can argue that the role of the counsellor is essentially facilitative. The actual diagnosis becomes secondary to the simple fact that the client is attending with some degree of psychological discomfort that is manifesting through a set of symptoms and behaviours that have been labelled as an 'illness'. Creating the therapeutic climate of empathic understanding, unconditional positive regard and authenticity creates a relational climate in which the client's own inherent capacity towards actualising fuller potential can become directed towards establishing a fresh sense of self that is liberated from the 'conditions of worth' that are all too often at the root of psychological discomfort.

Whether this liberation will be fully achieved in six sessions no one can actually know until the sessions have been completed. We do not have a crystal ball, and we cannot see into the future. We do not know how a particular person will respond to experiencing the facilitative climate offered by the person-centred therapist. It may be that the six sessions are a first step, but they may be necessary and sufficient for that particular person at that time to resolve the psychological difficulty that has become a problem. What is key here is that the emphasis is on the underlying experiencing of the client and not the outer symptoms. The latter can be thought of as the neon sign flashing to attract attention, saying that something needs attention. Here we have a distinct difference between the medical model and the person-centred in the therapeutic context. The former tends to treat conditions, the latter works with the whole person.

Imagine a wilting plant. We can spray it with some specific herbicide or pesticide to eradicate a perceived disease that may be present in that plant, and that may be enough. But perhaps the true cause of the disease is that the plant is located in harsh surroundings, perhaps too much sun, not enough water, poor soil, near other plants that it finds it difficult to survive near. Maybe by offering the plant a healthy environment that will facilitate greater nourishment according to the needs of the plant, it may become the strong, healthy plant it has the potential to achieve. Yes, the chemical intervention may also be helpful, but if the causes of the disease are environmental then it won't actually achieve sustainable growth.

The person-centred counsellor offers a facilitative climate such that the growth potential of the individual person can find expression in ways that the client finds fulfilling and satisfying. Even when six sessions may not be enough, at least some positive effects will be present and the client may be in a clearer position to decide what they wish to aim for in terms of their own lives and dealing with what has been disturbing them.

The client who has attended to deal with relational issues may realise that however much they might seek to modify their reactions to a demanding partner, the reality is that both need to change if the relationship is to continue in a fulfilling manner. So the counselling may not resolve the client's depression *per se*, but it could leave the client with a sense of direction and purpose that helps them to feel better about themselves because they can see something to work towards. Yes, they will continue to feel depressed, but may have recognised through the counselling process that the relationship had been attractive because they had been conditioned to seek a partner that reflected some introjected values from the client's childhood, but which essentially are not the values that the client holds to. The client may leave the counselling still experiencing symptoms of depression about the situation, but with a clearer intention to discuss the position openly with their partner, perhaps try couple counselling, maybe begin to build a greater life of their own based on the fresh sense of self and potentiality they are developing.

Person-centred counselling is not about symptom management or treatment for specific conditions. It is much more about offering a climate of relationship with someone which can induce shifts in the individual. The effect of this can be a lessening of the need for that person to experience discomforting symptoms and/or to pursue behaviours that are problematic or which are damaging to the individual or others.

Is it ethical to start counselling when there is a possibility that time limited may not be enough? Surely there is always this possibility, whatever the issue, because at the time the counselling begins, the counsellor and client may be quite unaware of deep-seated issues that lie beneath the surface and which have relevance to the presenting problem. The most innocuous problem – anxiety when out shopping, for instance – may track back through feelings of stress due to problems at home, which in turn are the result of having little confidence in a role at home because that person as a child experienced a home life of chaos and unpredictability and has introjected a belief that disorganisation is normal and that to be organised is therefore unsatisfying. This in turn, however, is linked to an experience of violence in the home, which the client has dissociated, and of feeling threatened in places where there is a lot of noise and uncertainty, and strangers who are too close for comfort.

The person-centred counsellor trusts that the client's tendency to actualise their potential will work within the context of the time available, and if deeper, underlying traumas are remembered and become present, then the client has the capacity to deal with them. The organism of the person is regarded as having fundamental intelligence and will maintain repression of memories where the person is not sufficiently able to deal with them. Where issues that the client wants more therapeutic support to address do arise, then there is need to refer that person on to other services.

We live in a world that believes that issues are like worms in a can, and when the lid is removed the client will be unable to contain them. The question we should ask is who decides to open the can of worms, and when? The non-directive aspect of person-centred counselling does not force the can open, it allows the client to open their own can should they so wish. The client may choose to press the lid back down, deciding that at that time in their life they would prefer to seek to cope with it and may need to seek strategies to achieve this. It may be that the client selects a particular worm representing one issue that they wish to work on. It may be that a large worm gets out and needs addressing, and referral on is required. Whatever happens, the key factor is that in person-centred counselling, the client's own process gives the counselling direction, not the ideas, goals or agendas of the counsellor or the referrer. The client knows they have a limited period of time and it is for the counsellor to trust the client's inherent capacity and potential as a person to use that time in whatever way they feel will be helpful. It is empowering of the client to take responsibility for themselves.

Counselling in a primary healthcare setting

Working in primary healthcare brings with it a whole host of issues that counsellors are advised to be prepared for. Many of these are dealt with in this book. My own experience has been interesting. There is a particular culture within primary healthcare. It can be quite frantic at times and the humour can sometimes seem difficult, then just as you think all is chaos you witness an emergency situation. A GP who is joking one moment is suddenly focused and present for a child who has been brought in looking very pale and sickly, then the next thing you hear is the receptionist being detailed to drop everything and call the ambulance. The primary healthcare environment is a very pressured, demanding and stressful one.

People consult their GP because they are unwell, and so the counsellor can naturally expect to be referred clients who may be struggling to come to terms with a distressing diagnosis, or with pain. Many referrals will be for mental, though more often emotional, health problems. These can range from depression and feelings of desperation and hopelessness through to anxiety states and stress associated with all kinds of causes: work, home, relationships. Depending on what has been agreed, given the service requirements of the surgery and the competence of the counsellor, clients may also be referred with drug or alcohol problems, suicidal tendencies, mild eating disorders. Such clients are unlikely to be referred where a rigid time-limited counselling service is being provided. Sometimes the client will have been prescribed medication, sometimes not. The counsellor needs an appreciation of the effects of medication, particularly those that are mood altering and which may limit the client's ability to experience feelings.

Some surgeries have dedicated counselling rooms, at other times the counsellor may be using a GP's consulting room or the nurses' room. These can contain all kinds of medical instrument that can be disturbing to the sensitive client, or the client who has experienced some form of medical trauma. Also, the client has a certain expectation and association with the environment. They may experience an expectation of the counsellor being prescriptive, simply because that is what they are used to in that setting.

Clients can experience a range of sensory challenges with primary healthcare (Bryant-Jefferies, 1999), so a little thought is needed. When a non-dedicated counselling room is being used for counselling, the counsellor needs to be aware of what is in the room. I was faced, well actually my client was faced, literally, with a life-size drawing of a skeleton on the back of the door, which local school-children had drawn for the surgery nurse. I hadn't noticed it until I closed the door after my client had walked in and sat down facing the door! There is also the smell to consider. A colleague of mine always takes an air freshener spray with him to freshen up the room. Posters on the walls can be disturbing for clients. Using a nurse's room where there are posters about the healthcare of babies may compound the difficulties for a client seeking counselling following a miscarriage.

GP surgeries are busy places, and rooms often have multiple uses. Storage can be a problem, with items kept in the room that is used by the counsellor. Always have a sign up on the door saying 'Please do not disturb, counselling in progress', particularly if you are using a room that is not dedicated to counselling. People are forever wanting to go into rooms because they have left something behind or are searching for a leaflet, a medical bag or the rubber gloves. The sign will help to stop this. Sometimes, however, access will be required if something in the room is urgently needed to treat someone. For instance, a nurse needing some equipment to treat a child experiencing an asthmatic attack had to come into a multi-user room where I was counselling.

Each counsellor may have their own system for taking referrals, or the surgery may have its own way of dealing with this. In my experience, the counsellor is the best person to allot appointments, otherwise they can be overwhelmed with referrals, all booked in with little scope for clients to be offered follow-up counselling sessions. This needs to be negotiated with the GPs and there needs to be clarity. The information to be included in the actual referral to the counsellor also needs to be agreed. How much history should the counsellor be given? What is relevant and what simply leaves the counsellor with a head full of knowledge about a client that is not relevant and may not be what the client would have wanted the counsellor to be aware of?

Note taking is an important factor. Counselling notes should be brief, factual and, if on paper, kept in a locked cabinet within the surgery. The key should be held by some responsible person within the surgery who understands the nature of counselling confidentiality – the senior partner, lead mental health GP or perhaps the practice manager. Some counsellors may also note on a slip of paper within the client's notes when a client has attended. It can help the GP to know that the patient they have referred is actually attending. This should be agreed with the client. However, many surgeries now keep notes electronically. It is important that the counsellor follows local protocols where they are working either for a primary care trust (PCT) or a mental health trust, both of which will have formulated protocols concerning the completion of, access to and retention of notes. The BACP (2000) has an information sheet entitled *Record Keeping and the Data Protection Act* and, at the time of writing, BACP is working on an information sheet on the topic of making notes.

Balancing the need to maintain confidentiality whilst working within the culture of a multidisciplinary team is important. Peter Jenkins (2002a) has written timely on this theme and on the impact of data protection law on access to a patient's health record, of which counselling notes from sessions within the NHS can be argued to form a part (2002b).

Language should also be considered, and not simply in the notes. The counsellor may be the only person in the surgery who sees 'clients', everyone else sees 'patients'. The words carry different meanings and a different emphasis. 'Patient' implies a person who requires treatment. The word 'client' can have more of a consultative feel about it. In the days of fundholding, I remember there being a move to encourage patients to be referred to as 'customers'. Thank goodness that has been dropped. The way I think of it is that I see *people* who are my *clients* and who are also *patients* of the surgery.

The need for patients to give informed consent to treatment is a development that has importance for the counsellor. Jenkins (2002b) indicates that 'informed consent, based on a legalistic model, requires the patient to have:

- access to relevant information, including risks and benefits
- capacity, or a sufficient level of understanding of the issues
- agreement to treatment being carried out'.

Emphasising the importance of *informed* consent, Jenkins indicates one possible solution to be a pre-therapy assessment session in which information is given to the client and informed consent obtained and documented. However, he also indicates that 'the exploration of consent needs to be seen as a continuing process, rather than a one-off event'. From a person-centred perspective, the initial assessment, if carried out by the counsellor, would be regarded as the start of therapy and the building of the therapeutic relationship.

Working in a GP surgery will give the counsellor a wealth of experience and will offer an opportunity for them to understand how primary healthcare works, and for other members of the primary healthcare team to appreciate the nature and particular discipline of counselling. It requires an openness, I believe, to collaborative working.

Having a supervisor with some experience of working in this environment can also be helpful, and some would argue is a necessity. Certainly, I have found it valuable to have supervisors with experience in this area, and in supervising clients who themselves work in GP surgeries and healthcare settings I have frequently drawn from my own experience when discussing issues that arise. It seems to me that it is a specialist environment and this needs to be fully appreciated and respected.

I also favour a collaborative approach, and I tend to describe this as a process of 'collaborative review'. Merry (2002, p. 173) describes what he terms 'collaborative inquiry' as a 'form of research or inquiry in which two people (the supervisor and the counsellor) collaborate or co-operate in an effort to understand what is going on within the counselling relationship and within the counsellor'.

This has been a brief introduction to what is a complex subject. Person-centred theory and its application in a time limited framework such as within primary healthcare continues to develop. A list of suggested reading on general person-centred theory and counselling within primary healthcare is included at the end of the book.

I would like to end this introduction by emphasising that *Time Limited Therapy in Primary Care: a person-centred dialogue* has been written, more than anything else, to offer the reader an *experience*. I hope you are affected by what you read and that it has a positive effect on your client work.

SESSION 1

Mandy had never been to counselling before. Her doctor had suggested she speak
to the surgery counsellor. She had come to the surgery the previous week feeling generally run down, finding it hard to motivate herself and just feeling
incredibly fragile. She didn't understand why she felt like this. She had always
been active and worked hard. OK, she had a demanding job as a marketing
executive, but she liked it; it made her feel alive. But recently it had all seemed
such a struggle. It all came to a head for her when she burst into tears one evening returning home on the train, and couldn't stop the tears. She had cried
driving home from the car park and for the rest of the evening. The next day
she had seen her GP and talked to her. She had felt better for that chat. Doctor
Hill had not prescribed anything, said she was reluctant to start a chemical
intervention when probably she needed a rest and some time to talk things
through with the counsellor.

So Mandy sat in the waiting room. She was aware that she was feeling anxious.
She knew that this wasn't like her. She had always felt confident, but now everything seemed an effort. She just felt so self-conscious sitting there. A couple
of minutes to go. As well as feeling anxious she was aware that there was a
tinge of relief. She also felt quite tense, her shoulders were stiff and she just
felt, well, generally tight. Felt odd, somehow. She didn't know what to expect.
She had heard things said about counselling, that it was all about making you
cry about your past. This had made her wonder if she really wanted this, but
the doctor had been quite persuasive, saying that the surgery counsellor was
a pleasant man called Martin, that many patients had benefited from counselling sessions with him. She had felt that Dr Hill had been genuine about this,
and she trusted her. She had helped her with a few minor problems over recent
years. Mandy heard her name being called and turned to where the voice was
coming from.

'Hi, I'm Martin. And you are Mandy?' Martin noticed the slightly anxious look on
the face of the woman who had turned towards him.

'Yes, thank you,' Mandy replied.

'Come on through. The counselling room is just along the corridor.'

Mandy followed Martin along the corridor. He stepped back and let her enter
the room first. It seemed pleasant enough, pale lemon/white walls, two

comfortable-looking chairs, a small table, a couple of prints on the walls. It felt quite a contrast to all the other rooms that she had been in at the surgery.

Rooms used for counselling in GP surgeries and healthcare settings generally vary a great deal. Sometimes it is a GP's room or a nurse's room. These are never ideal as the décor and the whole feel of the room is generally highly 'medicalised', conjuring up an expectation within the client of being given a specific 'treatment' by an 'expert'. This is not the nature of counselling, particularly person-centred counselling, which by its very nature is relational and which seeks to encourage a greater balance of power between client and therapist. Should the person being seen be thought of as 'a patient', 'a client' or as 'a person who happens to have a problem to resolve'? Language can so easily shape attitudes. The need to 'de-medicalise' the counselling environment can be so important.

When collecting a client from a waiting area in a surgery, the client has a right to feel that the reason she is there is confidential. Introducing yourself with 'Hello, my name is Martin and I am the counsellor' is inappropriate when other people are in the waiting area.

'So, Dr Hill has referred you and she has given me some background to what has happened. I understand things have kind of got on top of you and she felt that having some time to talk things through and explore what has happened and is happening for you would be helpful.'

Martin has deliberately kept it non-specific as he wants to leave it for Mandy to feel free to pick up on what is most imporant for her. His approach is 'non-directive', trusting that the client knows what they need to focus on. He also wants to be transparent, to ensure that his client is aware of what he already knows about her. In an approach that values the counsellor's congruence, there is a need to try and ensure that secrets are not being held. Martin is keen to encourage openness.

'Yes,' Mandy replied, 'but I'm not sure where to begin.'
'Not sure where to begin, sounds like there are a lot of different places you feel you could start from?'
'That's right.'
'OK. Can I check whether you have had counselling before?' Martin asked.
'No.'
'Would it help if I said something about it?' Martin sensed that Mandy was uneasy but he did not voice this. He knew that too much empathy of this kind early in a session can make clients feel unnecessarily uncomfortable and vulnerable.

'Yes, it would. I've heard different things but, well, some of it makes me feel apprehensive.'

'OK. Well counselling is an opportunity for you to talk through difficulties and for me to listen to you and help you to become more openly aware of yourself and to maybe make choices to help you feel more satisfied with your life. It's not that I am going to have answers, I actually believe that we all have more resources within ourselves than we often give ourselves credit for. I hope to help you feel able to talk about whatever you feel you want to air.'

'OK. That feels strange hearing you say that you are not going to have answers. I was hoping you'd tell me what was wrong and what to do.'

'It would be nice to be given answers, yes?'

Mandy nodded slowly. 'I just want to make sense of what is happening to me. I really am not sure where to start though.'

'OK, you want to make sense of things and I really hope that we can achieve that.' Martin was aware he hadn't clarified confidentiality. 'I do need to say that what is said here is confidential, and what I mean by that is that I would normally write a brief letter to the GP saying that we have had a first session, and what we plan to address and over how many sessions. I also update a card in the notes that confirms attendance at sessions and the focus of the session.'

'The GP said that there was a maximum of six sessions. How long is a session?' Mandy replied.

'Yes, it is a maximum of six sessions, and I generally see people for 50 minutes,' Martin responded, sensing that the number of sessions was an issue for Mandy. 'Does that leave you with any specific thoughts or feelings?' Martin always tried to offer the opportunity for clients to respond with thoughts or feelings. Counselling, in his view, was about engaging with the whole person and not simply directing them constantly into their feelings, or indeed only towards their thoughts as in more cognitive-behavioural approaches.

'Just seemed strange that there's a limit put on treatment before it has even started. But I guess there must be quite a demand.'

Martin could feel himself smiling. Nice one, he thought.

It is an important issue that counselling is often time limited, although not always to six sessions. Few other areas of NHS treatment are rationed in quite this way, and it is an area that needs resolving urgently. It sometimes seems that the 'quick-fix' culture has made its way into this important area of working. Some people do only require six sessions or fewer to work through an issue or difficulty, but others need longer. Martin knew that some surgeries offered counselling to an average of six sessions, which created greater flexibility. Unfortunately, this was not the service agreement that Martin had to adhere to, and he knew he resented it.

'It is strange, but it is what we have. At least we know the timescale we are working towards, and there are options for referral on should it become recognised by us both that longer-term work would be helpful.' Martin did not feel it appropriate to get into a philosophical discussion on the relative merits of six-session working. He hadn't actually finished highlighting confidentiality and what it meant, but it had seemed important to pick up on Mandy mentioning the six sessions.

'OK, we discuss that later if we need to?' Mandy asked.

'Yes. I need to say a little more about confidentiality. This is confidential. The letter to the GP does not go into detail over the content of the session. However, there are criteria for breaking confidentiality, for instance if you disclose anything that is indicative of intent to self-harm, including suicidal ideation and intent, intent to harm others or information concerning acts of terrorism. Also if you disclose anything that indicates harm to children, I then have a statutory obligation to breach confidentiality. Normally it will become obvious and we will talk about it should it arise.'

'That sounds heavy stuff. You have to tell everyone that?'

'It's good practice to do so. I think it is about being open and real. Confidentiality has its limits and I think it is important to be clear about this at the start.' Martin had initially felt uneasy at having to introduce this, particularly when clients often came through the door wanting to talk, or ready to release pent-up emotion in the first breath. But he knew he had to do this. He continued. 'And I need to say that counselling can be upsetting, it can release painful feelings or leave the person connecting with memories that are uncomfortable. It is not necessarily pain-free, although it doesn't have to be this way. It is important for you to feel clear about this as, in a very real sense, you have a right to know what you are consenting to.'

Providing clients with an information sheet about what to expect from counselling also helps ensure informed consent. This could be given by the counsellor, or by the referring GP.

Mandy nodded and thought about it. She didn't like the idea of connecting with painful memories, but then she thought that really her problems were about work and painful memories weren't really a factor. She was much more interested in sorting herself out and getting herself back to work again.

'OK. I consent, and I can see why you need to say all these things.' Mandy was feeling somewhat frustrated with all of this though, she had come along wanting to get on with talking about her problems, not to have to sit and listen to all of this.

Often clients do attend with this expectation, and this can create a tension. There is a strong argument to say that the GP should clarify the consent to counselling, allowing the counselling to begin from first contact, to ensure that the therapeutic relationship is being established from the start. But not all GPs are clear about counselling, and anyway, it would then be different to any other kind of referral for treatment. It is important for counsellors to develop their own style of conveying what needs to be said regarding confidentiality and clarity of what is being offered, so that informed consent is gained from the client.

Some counsellors will ask clients to sign a confidentiality agreement and a declaration of consent to counselling. Both can be helpful to clarify what has been agreed. However, it could be argued that both are being introduced from outside the client's frame of reference and that the client is being directed to sign them. This could therefore be regarded as contrary to the principles of person-centred counselling in which the client is encouraged, from the start, to make his or her own direction within the therapeutic relationship.

'I just want to find out why I feel so, I don't know, uptight about everything and have no energy to get on with things. I feel utterly deflated and bursting at the same time.'

'Yeah, deflated and bursting at the same time.' Martin kept to a simple straight reflection, as these words were spoken by Mandy with a lot of feeling. He said them slowly and deliberately.

'It's not like me. I like to live my life, get on with things. My job keeps me busy, and I really like it, but, oh, I don't know....' Mandy tailed off into silence and looked down.

Martin allowed the silence to run for a while. He could sense that this was a silence in which Mandy was connecting with her thoughts and feelings, and he wanted to respect this and allow her time before responding. He wanted to show his empathy for what she had been saying but now the priority felt it should be in holding the silence. After about 30 seconds he spoke quietly.

'You're not feeling like you. You like your busy job, but....' Again he allowed the silence that followed to be present.

'I do like my job and I feel good when I am moving around, getting sales, motivating my team, producing reports, I like the buzz. At least, I thought I did.'

'You thought that you did.'

'Yes, well I do.' Mandy took a deep breath. Yes, she did like her job, but she just felt that somehow she had had enough. All the rushing around, deadlines, targets, traffic jams. She looked up and met Martin's eyes.

'That sounded quite hesitant,' he responded, choosing to empathise with the way Mandy had spoken her words more than the words themselves.

'Yeah. It's just too much effort.' She could feel the tightness in her shoulders and she wanted to relax. It felt strangely good to feel that someone was listening to her. She hadn't really experienced that. It felt quite comfortable, although inside herself she could feel a dull ache somewhere inside her chest. She consciously made an effort to try and drop her shoulders and relax a little. She found it hard. 'Oh, I don't know.' She took another deep breath. Her eyes were beginning to brim with tears. She swallowed but said nothing. Her breathing returned to its normal rhythm. What is happening to me? she thought. I'm not going to start blubbing. She tried to compose herself. She felt strangely alone with her feelings, her anxieties, her sense of feeling overwhelmed by the demands of work, of not having time for herself, of not having space, of not knowing what to do, of feeling helpless, of feeling out of control. The thoughts, the feelings rushed in on her. She couldn't hold them back.

Martin felt a surge of compassion for Mandy. She looked so sad in that moment and somehow very small. He felt the presence of that deep sadness within himself. He wanted to do more than just hold the eye contact, so he tightened his mouth and nodded his head up and down, ever so slightly, and took a deep breath himself. He had learned with experience that taking a deep breath was actually a powerful therapeutic intervention for the client, often allowing them to do the same, which frequently led to emotional release of some kind.

> Martin's warmth is genuine, he is empathically in touch with his client and he is experiencing feelings within himself that are connected to this relational state. It is a powerful moment and he is right to voice what he senses as being present. The core conditions are all powerfully present and this will have a therapeutic impact on Mandy.

'I am sensing a lot of sadness, Mandy'. He used her name, it helped personalise the therapeutic and relational connection he was seeking to make with her.

'Yes.' Tears began to roll down Mandy's cheeks. Martin passed her a tissue, which she took gratefully and dabbed to her face. 'Yes.' Mandy could feel her body crumble. It was like all the energy that had been holding her so tight suddenly vanished. She felt weak and wobbly.

Martin said nothing, he trusted that Mandy needed to be experiencing whatever was happening for her. He believed strongly that offering a facilitative climate through empathy, congruence and unconditional positive regard would allow people to begin to risk being more open to themselves and allow that openness to find expression. He sensed that the tears were probably about more than the job, but he didn't want to push her into any disclosure. He trusted her own inner process to prompt her to do this if and when the time was right for her.

Mandy was feeling sad and she felt lost about her job, about everything. 'I do like my job, but somehow it doesn't seem so important any more.'

'Doesn't seem so important,' Martin responded, phrasing his empathic response with a slight questioning tone to his voice.

'It, oh I don't know, it somehow seems to be too much bother. I don't know. I mean, what's the point? What is the point? The company I work for isn't really interested in its staff – hire and fire. I suppose I've always known this, but it seems I'm more aware of it now. Seems like the way of the world – what price loyalty, huh?' Mandy let out a long sigh. 'I've been five years with the company. Five years.'

'Five years,' Martin replied.

Mandy breathed deeply and sighed again. 'I've had enough. But what can I do? I have a mortgage and bills to pay. God, I feel so trapped, so bloody depressed about it all.' The tears began again. 'What can I do?'

'You've had enough, you feel trapped and depressed, and you really want an answer to it all, yeah?'

'Yes, I can't go on like this. I can't go on like this.'

These straight, empathic reflections can read strangely as they are unusual in terms of normal conversation. Yet within a counselling environment they do communicate effectively to the client that they are being listened to and have been heard. While counselling is often described under the banner of 'talking therapies', the truth is that its power and effectiveness stem more from it being a 'listening therapy', but good listening is not passive.

Empathic responses allow the counsellor to check that he has heard correctly what the client is communicating and allow the client to feel heard and to hear her own words outside herself. The latter may lead the client to decide that the words she has used are not quite communicating what she wanted to say and she can then correct herself. This allows the client to more accurately define for herself what she is thinking, feeling and/or experiencing. It is particularly important that clients define their own experiences, encouraging self-refection and greater, more accurate, self-awareness.

'Can't go on like this,' Martin responded, deliberately speaking slowly so that Mandy had time for his reflection to be heard.

A silence followed. Martin respected it and allowed it to continue. Silences are times in which much can occur within a client and a relationship. It did not feel uneasy, although like many silences where upset is present, it was clearly bringing discomfort to Mandy. But he trusted that her experiencing of this discomfort in a room with a therapeutic companion would be helpful. He maintained his sense of warmth towards Mandy, his attention, while ensuring that he didn't stare (the nature of the therapist's eye contact can be warm or it can be invasive). He also sought to maintain his sensitivity towards his own experiencing, noting again that he was still carrying a sense that somehow there was more to this than the job, but he said nothing. If there was, it would be more therapeutically valuable for Mandy to make the connection and disclose it.

After a few minutes of silence, Martin felt he wanted to ensure that Mandy was aware of his presence, but he did not want to disturb what she was experiencing. He spoke softly, 'It is OK to just be with what you are feeling, no need to say anything unless you want to.'

Mandy nodded her head, almost imperceptibly. It felt good to know that there was someone out there listening and giving her attention. She had been quite lonely at times in recent years, since her mother had died. That was five years ago now. She had been upset at the time, but had got on with things. It had been around the time that she had changed jobs. She was aware that her thoughts were moving away from work and her sense of feeling unable to go on. She could now see her mother's face very clearly in her mind's eye. Smiling at her. She could almost hear her saying, 'It's OK Mand' (she always called her Mand, never did know why), 'It's OK.' She could feel her throat drying and her heart was pounding. The tears began again, but they felt hotter now.

'Oh God, I miss her.' The words came out leaving Martin unsure who Mandy was talking about. Should he ask, or stay with the feeling. He stayed with the feeling. No doubt the who would be revealed later.

'You miss her so much.' Martin spoke softly.

The tears were flowing from Mandy's eyes now. She put her head in her hands and rested her elbows on her knees. She hadn't cried like this since, well, she hadn't cried like this at all before. She could feel pain in her chest as she sobbed, finally taking her hands away from her face and reaching out for another tissue. She took a deep breath and blew the air out of her mouth. She looked up at Martin, and swallowed. 'My mother.'

Martin nodded, it really didn't need a verbal response. However, he felt a strong sense of the importance that Mandy's mother had been to her. He voiced it, not as a question – it would have been silly, of course she would have been important. The tears, the sobbing showed that. 'She was really important to you,' and after a short pause he added, 'and you miss her.'

Mandy's head went back into her hands and she began sobbing again. She drew in deep breaths but could not stop the flow this time. She lost all sense of time. She felt this huge ache in her body, in her stomach and reaching up into her chest and her heart. The back of her throat burned and her head felt strangely heavy.

Minutes passed. Martin sat and wondered should he reach out to Mandy.

> When is it appropriate for a counsellor to initiate physical contact with a client during distress? This is a huge issue. It is exacerbated when the counsellor is the gender of the client's preferred sexual attraction. One good rule to apply is to consider whether there is hesitancy. If in doubt, the answer is probably don't. However, where it feels like a genuine and natural human response, then it is more likely to be accepted as being a genuine human response expressive of warmth and unconditional positive regard. But the counsellor must know themselves well enough to be able to distinguish their motivation. In this instance, it is a first session, which, for some counsellors, will mean that they are probably less likely to initiate physical contact in the form of, perhaps, touching the client's arm, but not all will feel this way.

Martin did a quick reality check. What were his feelings at this time? He felt compassion. He felt care and warmth towards another human being who was clearly in deep distress. It felt clear, there were no other thoughts encroaching.

But it was a first session, he really did not know much about Mandy. He could voice his dilemma, but that might just take Mandy away from what she was experiencing. He could hear the words of a trainer from his past in his mind, 'When in doubt, keep it simple.' He could feel a kind of inner smile.

'Mandy, if it would help to have someone touch your arm. . . .'

Oh yes, Mandy thought, it feels horrible in here. She took her left hand away from her face and reached out. She felt Martin's warm touch. And she felt the surge of hurt inside herself again and she forgot his touch as the tears increased again. She returned her left hand to her face instinctively. All she could feel was this deep hurt, an ache that just would not go away. It was like she was that ache, there was nothing of her extending beyond it. She was not really thinking, she was just being this ache, this deep hurt, or the ache was being her.

Time passed and Martin sat holding his feelings of warmth for Mandy. She was clearly hurting so much and he really admired her for being able to bring these feelings into the room. He also knew that probably the dam was just waiting to burst, but maybe the way he had been at the start of the session had been enough for something inside her to recognise that it was safe to let these feelings out. It was nice to think it was him being a good counsellor, but he knew that sometimes people were so keyed up and ready to release, that any pleasant face indicating signs of caring in the room would have been enough.

These thoughts were only momentary. Martin kept his focus on Mandy, who was beginning to go quiet, the sobs less frequent. After a couple more minutes had passed she began to rub her eyes and reached out for another tissue. Her eyes were quite red and her collar was damp where the tears had dropped.

She took another deep breath and blew it out, looking up at Martin as she did so. 'I wasn't expecting any of that,' she said, shaking her head somewhat in disbelief.

'Really took you by surprise?' Martin responded.

'Yeah, that hurt. That really hurt. But somehow it feels easier now.' She blew out another long breath.

'So much hurt, but easing a bit now, yeah?'

'I feel quite light-headed.' Mandy reached out to the glass of water on the table. She took a few sips and replaced it. 'Have I been carrying this around for five years?'

'Five years?' Martin responded, hoping for some clarification.

'My mum died five years ago, just before the change of job to my current one. I didn't cry much at the time. I was, well, I suppose I was too busy. I was upset and I did cry, and friends were really supportive, but I never felt anything like I did just now.' Mandy was still looking shocked by what had happened.

'It can be quite a shock to experience that strength of feeling and hurt, it can leave you quite disorientated.'

Mandy nodded her head.

'You'll need to look after yourself when you leave. People can feel very sensitive after this kind of experience. Take it quietly if you can.' Martin was aware that this was coming straight from his own frame of reference and while he did not want to create an expectation in Mandy, he knew from experience how powerful these kind of experiences can be.

'Yes. I'm actually meeting up with a friend for lunch, a good friend, so I think that will help.'

Martin was aware that time had passed and there were only ten minutes or so of the session left. 'Mandy, we have about ten minutes left. How do you want to use the time? And we also need to agree whether you want to continue with counselling, as we have not talked about that.'

'Yes, I do want to carry on. Definitely. I have to get myself sorted. I'm not sure how but I do need to get myself together.' The words sounded quite strong and affirming.

'You sound strong when you say that, as though you are really affirming it to yourself.'

Empathic responses are not necessarily in response to what the client is saying. The tone of voice can usefully be reflected back to the client. It also shows the client that you are listening beyond the words, that you are not simply reflecting back what she has said. Empathy is more than reflection. It is certainly not a technique to be applied for a specific purpose. It is simply the allowing of the client to feel heard, understood and related to another human being. In this instance, Martin has communicated his experience of the presence of strength and self-affirmation in the way Mandy had been speaking. It enables Mandy to acknowledge the presence of these qualities, and to then risk acknowledging a less secure part of herself as well. She brings parts of herself together and feels more whole as a result.

'Yes, I somehow feel stronger, although I feel wobbly as well. I feel different. I think I need time to make sense of all of this. How often do you want to see me?' Mandy asked.

'Before I answer your question, I want to acknowledge that I hear you wanting to take time to make sense of what you are experiencing.' Martin felt himself nodding and a phrase came to mind from somewhere, 'and it is so easy to forget to take time for ourselves'. He could feel a smile as he heard himself say these words. He knew they were partly for his own benefit, yet somehow they did feel the right thing to say.

Sometimes a response to a client can seem to contain aspects of the counsellor, but they may still be appropriate for the client to hear. Again, the safeguard is that the counsellor is experiencing connection to the client in that moment.

Mandy took a deep breath. 'Time for myself. Yes.' She sat silently for a moment. 'Yes, I have to work at that. It was good to be reminded of that, and I felt anxious at the thought of it too.' She nodded her head slowly and smiled. 'OK, so how often?'

'Well, weekly or fortnightly is what I can offer, and another five sessions maximum. What do you feel would be helpful to you in terms of frequency of contact?'

'Weekly, particularly as I am off work at the moment and it might be difficult when I return. No, I want to get on with this. Though quite what I do next time I do not know.' Mandy felt quite overwhelmed by what had happened, yet something instinctively told her that this was where she needed to be. She had never experienced that depth of feeling, or experienced someone to be so attentive and caring to her. And a man as well! The kind of man she could do with. That had felt good. She didn't say any of this, though.

'OK, so weekly, and is this time and day OK?' Martin asked.

'Fine.'

'OK. So I will write a short note to Dr Hill. Do you mind my mentioning that as well as focusing on your current feelings associated with work, we will also be addressing the feelings linked with your mother?'

'Dr Hill knows about my mother dying, but yes, mention that it has come up here. How much do you tell her?'

'I could draft it out now if you like so you know what I am saying.' Martin was more than happy to offer this. It provided an opportunity to reflect on the session and to capture it succinctly. It also ensured that what was said was agreed by them both. He knew of situations where clients had accessed notes and complained about what had been said.

'No, just tell me what you plan to say.' Mandy felt she could trust Martin and besides, there hadn't been anything expressed in the session that Dr Hill was unaware of.

'OK, I'll say we met up today for the first session, that we have agreed to five more counselling sessions, and that while we will be addressing the reasons for your low mood and motivation, we will also be addressing the effect of the loss of your mother.'

'Fine. I'll see you next week then. Thanks for listening. I'm still surprised by that session. Think I need a stiff drink with my lunch!'

Martin heard the alarm bell go off in his head. A reasonable response for Mandy to make, but he also knew that alcohol use could become problematic when it was linked to anaesthetising feelings. Was this how Mandy coped with emotional discomfort? He didn't know. Anyway, he let it pass. It was his stuff. The session was ending.

Towards the end of sessions, clients can say things and the counsellor, aware that the client is perhaps preparing and adjusting to return to the world outside the counselling room, and relaxing himself, can say something that affects the client adversely, particularly if it has a negative component to it. It may be said humorously, but the counsellor cannot be sure how the client will take it. This end-of-session transition phase can be extremely significant. It can also be extremely therapeutic because the manner of parting is the final impression that is made upon the client before she leaves to spend the week making sense of what the counselling was all about.

'OK. You know your way out. Oh, and I should have said, if for any reason you cannot make an appointment, can you call and let the surgery know?'

'Sure.'

'Thanks. I hope today has been helpful.' Martin said this with genuineness. He had enjoyed the session and was hopeful that it had been helpful. 'See you next week.'

Mandy left the room and went outside. She felt lighter somehow, as if a weight had been lifted. She was still amazed by what had happened and while part of her wanted to think about it and reflect on the experience, she was aware of the time and she had that lunch date to get to. So she hurriedly headed off to her car and drove off towards the restaurant where she was meeting her friend. Yes, she thought it had been helpful, although she couldn't quite pin down exactly how.

Martin sat for a while after the session. It had been emotionally draining for him. So much emotion present in the room, so much hurt. It had been palpable. And it still felt very present, although he was sitting there on his own. Thank goodness he had a short break before the next client, he would need those 15 minutes. He was aware of his usual anxieties over whether six sessions would be long enough. Yet he felt that in this instance they might be, and if they were not, it would hopefully be clearer by the end of the final session what else Mandy might need to do to feel able to move on in her life. She wasn't the first client to have come to a grinding halt in her work and then discover that beneath this were unresolved feelings from the past. It was often the case. He got out his file and wrote up his notes. He believed in keeping notes brief and to the point, with emphasis on facts and content. He did not write up any of his thoughts about process in the notes. He had his own personal journal that he used to track his own process in life. He never referred directly to clients in that, only to his own associated feelings and thoughts.

Letter to GP

Dear Dr Hill,

To let you know that I saw Mandy today. She has highlighted the stress of her job, and her struggle to feel motivated in the way that she is used to.

In the session she released a lot of emotion in relation to the loss of her mother.

We will be addressing the reasons for her low mood and motivation and also the effect on her of the death of her mother. It may be that other factors arise as Mandy explores her thoughts and feelings.

I shall be seeing Mandy weekly for the usual five more sessions.

Yours sincerely,

Martin Jones
Counsellor

Client case notes

New client, aged 36. Lives alone. Symptoms of depression, low motivation associated with work. Busy and demanding job which she has held for five years. During the session client released pent-up emotion associated with her mother's death five years ago. Death occurred prior to the new job. Client indicated that she had not experienced or released the degree of emotion and hurt I witnessed today. Agreed to weekly contact. Client aware of, and has agreed to, limits of confidentiality, has voiced consent to counselling and to contents of letter to her GP.

Points for discussion/action

- What other factors need to be taken into account in terms of the appropriateness of the room and environment when counselling in a GP surgery?
- Is there anything else that could have been mentioned by the counsellor at the start of the session?
- What are your feelings and thoughts towards physical contact with a client during a cathartic release?
- How would you introduce confidentiality issues in this setting?
- Mandy is well known to the GP. If she was not, would you write a different letter to her?
- Critically evaluate the session. Did Martin stay within the client's frame of reference? When did he voice congruent experiencing and was this helpful and appropriate?
- Make you own clinical notes of this session.

SESSION 2

When Martin arrived at the surgery Dr Hill caught him in the corridor. 'I'm glad you saw Mandy last week. I'm not surprised about her mother, especially as she had such a strange upbringing, you know – that period of fostering.'

'Shit,' thought Martin, 'I didn't need to know that. I'm getting stuff that the client isn't aware of me knowing.' He knew he had to say something to the GP straight away. 'I appreciate your wanting me to know this, and had it been in the referral letter then it would have been something I would have been able to have made the client know I was aware of. However, it makes it difficult when I pick up information once I have started seeing someone. So I will need to let the client know when I see her today that I am aware of this. I know that generally this information is helpful, and in a way it is, but the way I work is to let the clients disclose what they feel they need to disclose in their own time. And where information has been made available at the start through the referral process then I do like to make it visible. Helps to encourage openness, I think. So, I hope you don't mind me saying this, but that's counselling.'

Confidentiality within a GP surgery is obviously important. However, the meaning that a counsellor might ascribe to confidentiality is likely to be at variance with that of the GP or other healthcare professional. Primary healthcare works at its effective best when information is shared. However, that sharing must be on a need-to-know basis and not a 'want to know'. Staff will have confidentiality agreements written into the contracts. However, for the counsellor, it is important the confidentiality of what is disclosed and transpires within the session remains confidential to counsellor and client, except for the counsellor's supervisor. Disclosures will be passed on to the GP where it is in the client's interest and with her consent. There may, however, be times when confidentiality will be breached, for instance if a client is indicating suicidal intent with a clear plan but not wanting anyone else to know. The counsellor is part of a healthcare team and is most effective when he integrates. This has the added advantage of providing an opportunity to educate other healthcare professionals as to the nature of counselling.

Martin was waiting when Mandy arrived. She was on time. He went out into the waiting area and invited her into the counselling room. They settled down.

Mandy started speaking straight away before Martin had a chance to say anything about what Dr Hill had told him.

'I feel so much better after last week. I felt a little woolly when I left, but having then met with my friend and talked about things, particularly what had happened in the session, and had a few laughs as well, you know, I really felt I moved on.' Mandy was smiling. She really felt a lot better and had really begun to get on with organising a few things in her life. She still had another week signed off from work and had decided she was going to make the most of the time.

'So, feeling much better after last week, and feeling you have moved on,' Martin responded deciding to stay with Mandy and not introduce anything about the fostering.

'Yes.'

'So, how do you want to use the time today?'

Mandy had given it some thought and she felt she actually wanted to spend time focusing on her job and what she should do.

'I'd like to discuss my job, or at least the pros and cons of staying or leaving, and just what I feel about it. Although I do feel more energised I also know that I have not been happy there and I'm really still wondering if I want to go back to it.'

Martin wondered about reflecting all that Mandy had said but decided it would sound stupid. He decided to keep it minimal and just repeat the last few words.

'So, still wondering if you want to go back to it.'

'Yes, it has been such a big part of my life these past five years, and I have some good friends there, but it's hard work, long days and I never seem to have much time for myself.'

'Mhmm,' Martin responded, wanting to acknowledge he was listening but without interrupting Mandy's flow.

'I just think there is more to life than working, particularly when all I seem to get is pressure, pressure, pressure. I think I've had enough but I guess I'm not completely sure. It would be a big step to leave. I feel kind of trapped, but I know I'm not. I can make the choice to leave, but what then? Wind up in the same situation somewhere else? Better the devil you know and all that.' Mandy could feel anxiety rising as she spoke. The thought of going back to work was not an attractive one. But . . . the alternative was a big step.

Martin had noticed the anxious look on Mandy's face as she spoke and decided rather than show only empathy for her words, he would also mention her expression.

'So, pressure, pressure, pressure. Feeling trapped but better the devil you know. And I can't help noticing that as you spoke you seemed to look more and more anxious.' Martin could relate to what Mandy was saying from his own experience. He had felt that way before deciding to train as a counsellor. But he was able to put this memory aside. It was not pressing but it did make him realise he had to be sure to listen to what Mandy was telling him and not make assumptions based on his own experience.

Are counsellors who have had similar experiences to their clients more likely to be helpful, or those who have not? Some clients want to speak to someone who understands through what they themselves have experienced, yet for others it does not matter. Perhaps it depends more on the counsellor's personality. Feeling a strong, curious interest in clients and wanting to be a companion to them as they try to resolve whatever is troubling them is perhaps what matters. The person-centred counsellor is not there to have the answers, but rather to help clients openly explore their own feelings and thoughts in order to discover or formulate their own solution.

'I think in an ideal world I would leave, but not before I had something else to go to.'

Martin could feel an instant response come to mind as he felt himself drawn to wonder what an ideal world meant for Mandy.

'So, I am curious, what would an ideal world look like?'

Mandy sat for a moment and thought about it. That was a good question. What would an ideal world look like? 'Well, I suppose it would be a world in which I knew what I was going to do next.'

'A world in which you knew your next step.' Martin slightly altered the wording in his empathic response. Sometimes it could be a bit much for clients to hear only their own words coming back at them, and it didn't seem vital to use the exact words on this occasion.

A world in which I would know my next step. Mandy thought about this. No, that was too simple. She looked at Martin and said, 'No, not just that. No, an ideal world wouldn't just be about my work. It would be about where I lived as well. Where I live, well, it's an expensive area and I have a small house. But it is busy, the main road passes outside and there always seems to be traffic these days. I've been there for three years and when I first moved there it seemed right, with good transport links and closer to the office. Now, I'm not so sure.'

'So there were advantages when you moved there, or so you felt at the time, but now you are not so sure.'

'Yes, I'm really not sure, but I've done so much work there, well not so much on the house, but the garden I have really created myself. It's only small, but I have created a Mediterranean-style environment and it feels really good. Well, when I have time to sit in it, which doesn't seem very often these days. You know, this past week I think I spent more time sitting and appreciating that garden than I have in the whole of the last year.'

Martin kept to an empathic reflection of the last few words to allow Mandy to continue, '. . . whole of the last year.'

'Well, maybe not the whole of the last year, but it certainly does feel like it. I've been so busy, it feels like I've lost sight of something important. I think I've lost sight of some very basic things in my life, such as simple pleasures and having time to enjoy things. I'm always in such a rush. It's so stressful.' Mandy could feel rising irritation with herself as she said this.

'So the busy-ness has caused you to lose sight of simple things that you can enjoy.' How many clients had Martin seen who had spent years as 'human *doings*' before finally burning out and realising they needed to get back to becoming 'human *beings*'.

Many people experience the symptoms of stress and often it has a simple origin. Either they feel they have to do something that they no longer want to do, or they are being asked to do something they do enjoy, but not for 12 hours or more a day. In either case, the person feels unable to say 'no', feels out of control and overloaded.

'Yes, I need to make changes. In my ideal world I would have time; time for *myself*, time to do the things that *I* really want to do.' Mandy took a deep breath as she finished. It felt good saying these things, and also to have someone who seemed to be taking her seriously, but how could she make them happen?

'Changes. Time for yourself, time to do the things that you really want to do.' Martin emphasised two words, 'yourself' and 'you'. He wasn't sure exactly why he had showed particular empathy for those two words, but as Mandy had said them they had seemed to stand out. Maybe she had said them herself with a little more emphasis, he wondered. Anyway, no sense in dwelling on that, he noticed Mandy smiling.

As Mandy heard her words repeated back to her she could feel a surge of energy inside and her fists clenched seemingly without any conscious prompting. Yes, she thought, yes, time for me. She smiled.

As well as noting her smile, Martin had also seen her tightening her fists. He didn't want to say anything which might cause her to unclench them. He had noted how often commenting on body language can simply stop the movement that has been noted and the flow of experiencing that is behind the body movement. He wanted Mandy to stay with it. He responded with a deep breath and making a point of clenching his own fists.

Mandy smiled. 'Yes,' and she tightened her fists, 'I need some time for me in my life and I will find it. I feel more energy thinking about it.'

'Time for you. Feeling more energy. Feels good, huh?' Martin responded, relaxing his fists but wanting to help Mandy hold herself in her feelings as she experienced them.

'Yes. I'm amazed how strongly I feel. I mean, I realise work had got on top of me but I hadn't realised how strongly I was feeling about wanting more time for me.' Mandy was genuinely surprised, it showed on her face.

'You really look surprised about that.'

'I am. So, part of what I need is time for me.' She took a deep breath and sighed slightly. 'But I've got some decisions to make, and the first one is work. I go back next week, well, that is if I don't get another certificate from the GP. Part of me feels that I don't want to go back just yet, another part feels that it would be dishonest. So I'm not sure. What do you think?' she asked, looking Martin in the eyes.

'Sounds like you really are unsure what to do about work next week. My feeling is that you are the best person to know your own needs.'

'I'm really not sure. I suppose I might feel different about work now, although I know that isn't really likely. Same job. Same people. Same organisation. Same deadlines and targets. Yet I also know that it gives me a buzz, a kind of energy, and I'd miss that. When I'm out on the road either heading for a presentation or visiting team members, I feel great.' Mandy was thinking of those occasions when she was driving on an open road and felt a sense of freedom somehow.

'You really are in touch with both negative and positive experiences.' Martin deliberately ensured he made this comment voicing the negative and positive in the same order that Mandy had disclosed them. It meant she was less likely to be directed back into the negative, having ended her last sentence on a positive note, but he had let her know that he had heard both aspects of what she was saying.

'Yes, and I know I hate the pressure, but somehow I seem to thrive on it as well. Makes me feel alive. I love being busy, you know. But recently I was getting so tired, so fed up. Just couldn't be bothered any more. If I go back I want to feel sure I'll be able to continue feeling good, and maybe I'll experience it all differently.' Mandy sort of felt this was realistic but she had her doubts.

'So, will you be able to maintain your good feeling and will you experience work differently?'

'Yes. I think I want to go back, but I'm going to make sure I take the time to continue coming here as well. I feel I need to think things through not just short term but in the longer term as well. It would be good to look at whether I really want to stay in this job and maybe I'll know that more clearly once I go back and see how I feel about it. I'll have had three days back before I see you next week, if it is the same time, same day, and so I'll have something to go on. I think I need to leave thinking about the job just at the moment until then, is that OK?'

'OK, so wait and see how you react to going back to work, and then we explore whatever needs exploring next time, yes?' Martin could feel as he said this that he wasn't at all convinced that such a quick return to work was a good idea. He could sense Mandy's enthusiasm, which seemed to have emerged very strongly given that not so long ago she seemed to be in real doubt. He wondered how much she could trust this strength of feeling, but he was not here to question or undermine what she felt.

'Yes. Now I'm not sure what to talk about. Maybe I should go.' Mandy didn't really want to go, but she kind of felt awkward not knowing what to say next. She also wanted Martin to say he wanted her to stay. She liked him. He listened. He seemed to pay attention to her and, well, she liked it.

'So, nothing comes to mind, and you feel that you want to head off.' There was something that felt awkward for Martin. It didn't feel quite right. He felt as though he was hearing words but they didn't seem to ring true. He couldn't put his finger on it. He had had clients before who suggested they leave early because they felt that they had nothing more to say, and sometimes this was OK, and at other times it led back into another topic. But this felt different somehow. He really felt that Mandy was saying one thing but meaning something else.

These situations arise in counselling. The counsellor has a profound sense that something is not quite as it seems, but it is indistinct. Here, Mandy is attracted to Martin, but is not disclosing this. She is saying one thing but secretly hoping for a different outcome. Martin is fortunately sufficiently self-aware to recognise something is not quite right and he will trust his sensing. This situation becomes difficult when the counsellor blindly slips into small talk with the client, losing focus and becomes drawn into an incongruent state. He would be incongruent because he is present as a counsellor but would begin to start behaving outside of his role and professional boundary with sufficient self-awareness that he was doing this.

The need for counsellors to achieve a certain degree of self-awareness is important. This may be developed through therapy, but this is not the only method for people to get to know themselves. Meditation can also aid this, as can in-depth discussions with friends. New experiences that challenge a person's concept of themselves can also serve to enhance self-awareness and authenticity.

The room went quiet and it felt increasingly awkward. Mandy continued to smile. Martin felt that he had to say something, something did not feel right here.

'Mandy, I'm not sure what has happened here, but I kind of sense that you are saying you should go, and yet my sense is that you actually want to stay.'

Mandy could feel her face flushing. Shit, she thought. 'Phew, it's hot in here, can we open a window or something?'

Martin didn't feel any heat in the room, but he had noticed Mandy flush. He sensed it as a diversion but he decided to open the window anyway while maintaining his focus.

'There, maybe some fresh air will be good.'

'Thanks,' Mandy replied.

'You don't really want to go, do you?' Martin did not add his curiosity as to what this was about as he felt that would be too confrontational. He wanted Mandy to explore what was happening at her own pace.

'No, I don't, but I also don't know what to talk about.'

'So, you don't want to go but you don't know what to talk about.' Martin kept it to a straight reflection. He wanted to keep his responses simple and to the point so that clarity might emerge.

'No, I don't want to go.' She hesitated, and then took a deep breath and continued. 'Martin, you were so good to me last week. No one has ever listened to me like that, well no man has, and it felt good. It felt steadying, solid.' She put her head in her hands. 'Oh God, what am I saying?'

'What are you saying, Mandy?' This felt like a very important moment, the room had suddenly gone very still and the atmosphere had changed. It felt very quiet and intense. Martin did not know what Mandy was going to say, but it seemed as though it was going to be important.

'I need a tissue.'

Martin handed her the box, which had been left under the table. Mandy removed one and pressed it against her face.

'You really seemed to care. I felt good. But I think I felt confused as well. I left here not sure what I was feeling, but I know I felt positive and seemed to be walking a little taller. But I was confused.' She began to cry. The room was silent apart from the sound of Mandy's short breaths as she struggled, and failed, to hold back the tears that were welling up in her eyes. Minutes passed.

Martin sat with his whole attention towards Mandy. He was aware of being unclear as to what had happened for Mandy. But he respected her right to silence and to be with her own feelings and thoughts at this time. He had heard her saying that she felt he had really seemed to care and that it had left her confused. She had said that she had left feeling positive but that confusion had remained. What was she confused about, he wondered? He brought himself back to Mandy, aware he had drifted into his own thoughts.

Mandy could feel a deep sadness inside herself again, but it was not the same as she had experienced the previous week. This was different and she couldn't quite distinguish why. She raised her head as though to look towards the ceiling but kept her eyes closed, taking a deep breath and letting it back out again, inflating her cheeks as she blew the air back out.

Martin was aware that the tears had stopped and he decided to wait and let Mandy say whatever she felt she needed to say in her own time. Just at that moment there was a sudden sound of raised voices outside the room in the corridor, which shattered the atmosphere in the counselling room. There was some heated discussion, and while the words were indistinguishable, it was enough to jar Mandy away from her feelings and Martin away from his focus on Mandy.

'Sorry about that. Felt as though it just cut across what was happening in here and for you.' Martin felt angry and knew it was on his face. He shook his head a little.

This kind of disturbance happens and the counsellor needs to be prepared to deal with it, to reassure the client and to allow her time to recover from the shock. And it can be quite a shock. One minute the client is centred in her feelings, the next moment she is jarred back into the room. It is important to be calm and acknowledge what has happened and allow the client to feel able to voice her reaction if she wishes to before encouraging the session to proceed.

Counsellors are encouraged to put signs up on the door to indicate that the room is in use and that they should not be disturbed. This is particularly so where the surgery does not have a dedicated counselling room, and the counselling is being offered in a room used by a nurse or perhaps a GP. Having someone burst into a counselling session can be shocking for the client, who may, in that moment, have connected with some deep hurt or be approaching some significant insight. It can all be swept away, and it can then take time for the client to feel confident that it won't happen again.

Mandy could see the anger on Martin's face. She didn't feel angry, but she did feel shaken by it. 'I was well away and then suddenly I was back here. I'm still collecting my thoughts. My heart is thumping.' She swallowed and looked down.
'Take your time,' Martin replied, 'take your time.'
Mandy was grateful for that. It had been a shock. The sadness had begun to subside but she had been feeling very sensitive and had felt herself jump when she first heard the voices. After about half a minute she looked up. 'I was feeling sad. It was what I had been saying and then I suddenly had this wave of sadness hit me.'
'A wave of sadness?' Martin reflected back but with a hint of questioning.
'Yes. It was as if I realised that no one had ever really been there for me like you were last week. No one has ever cared enough to listen to me, really listen to me. I felt very sad and very alone. Well, sort of alone. It was strange. I felt I wasn't alone in this room, but I somehow felt alone inside myself.' Mandy could feel herself going quiet and the sadness welling up again.
'No one has cared enough...,' Martin replied but did not get a chance to finish his sentence as Mandy had dissolved back into tears again.
'I'm sorry. I didn't mean to start crying again. I'm sorry.'
'No need to be sorry, Mandy, no need to be sorry.' Martin spoke as gently as he could, not wanting to disturb Mandy in her release of feelings.

Is Martin at risk of communicating non-acceptance of Mandy's need to feel sorry for crying again? Or is this an acceptable response, affirming that she has permission to cry if she wants or needs to?

'I just find it so hard, being like this, having someone giving me time, being there, here. Oh I don't know. It's confusing me.' She took a sharp breath and let it back out immediately. 'I am so confused.'
It didn't feel right to just reflect it. Martin decided to offer Mandy the opportunity to explore it a little more. He spoke softly. 'What are you confused about, Mandy?'
'I haven't had many relationships with men. Somehow, I've always been too busy to really get involved very much. Always been too busy – story of my life, huh? I just suddenly felt sad that here I am at 36, sitting here with a counsellor and suddenly realising this is the first time a man has really listened to me or paid attention to me, really paid attention to me. It's confusing. I mean, I don't know how to react, I really don't. I feel ... I guess I don't know what I feel. Am I making any sense here? I must sound crazy. Maybe that's what I am, going crazy.' Mandy felt desperate.
Martin heard the desperation in her voice. He felt he should reassure her that she was not crazy, yet he was also aware that this was what Mandy was feeling and wanted him to hear. 'What I am hearing is that you have never had a man really listen to you and that you are confused as a result of my paying you attention last week when you were in so much distress, and again today. It has left

you wondering if you are making any sense, if you are going crazy.' Martin could appreciate the confusion. When you encounter a new experience – and he was unclear what had occurred in Mandy's path that had left her bereft of this experience – it can be normal to be confused.

'Not just the attention. I felt you really cared.'

'I do care.' Martin heard the words come out before he could think about this response. 'I care about your wellbeing. I don't like people being in distress but I know that it is often a necessary part of counselling and coming to terms with deep hurt. Yes, I care.' It was after he had said this that the thought struck him that maybe he should have responded by saying something like, 'You felt cared for.' But he hadn't – supervision issue, he thought. Did I need to tell Mandy I cared? Did I need to then qualify it? Who was I telling her for, me or her? I need to talk this through with my supervisor. And I need to be just a bit more sensitive to my own reactions.

Sometimes the counsellor can find himself into a response to something that the client has said and then realise that he is explaining himself and knows that instead of being there for the client, the client is now listening to him. Generally, such occurrences do need talking through with a supervisor. The counsellor needs to understand where he is coming from in these situations so that his self-awareness is raised and if there is an unresolved issue behind it, that it can be identified and dealt with either in supervision, if that seems appropriate, or in personal therapy if more in-depth work is required.

However, perhaps it needs to be openly explored in the session with the client as well. Sometimes taking an issue to supervision is a 'safe' response, the more challenging one is to own it in the session. The reality is, Martin cares about Mandy, but he has been left feeling uncomfortable with his experience.

Martin decided to say what he had now thought of saying, 'You felt cared for.' This time he did not voice it as a question, but rather as a statement.

Mandy had turned to look out of the window and she seemed to be somewhat distant. Martin did not disturb her. She turned back. 'Sorry, miles away. I was looking at that tree, thinking how strong it looked, and then I noticed the small one next to it. So vulnerable-looking. I started to think that I kind of saw myself as that strong tree, but now, well, now I'm feeling more like the smaller one. The smaller one. . . .' Her words tailed off into a silence.

Martin reflected back her last words, 'the smaller one'.

'All on its own.' A silence followed. 'That was me. All on my own. I was fostered out when I was four. Don't remember too much about it but I know I had an unhappy time. My mother couldn't cope, well no, the truth is that she wouldn't cope. My father had left, they weren't married and she felt she had to build a career for herself – she was a researcher, scientific, and had decided to take time out to bring me up, but then my father left. She couldn't do this and be there for me. I stayed with my grandmother some of the time, but I also had time with foster parents. I was with them first, then with my grandmother, before returning back home. I didn't get back to living with my mother fully until I was about seven. I saw her and we had holidays together and weekends, but I guess it was confusing in a way. Everyone was good to me, but I felt on my own. I felt different.'

'All on your own, feeling different,' Martin replied, not worrying about all the information and keeping to what Mandy had experienced, was experiencing now perhaps, in herself.

'Yeah. I think I must have felt as though I was everyone's problem, you know? That's how it seemed. Just felt passed around. It got better later, but my mum was still busy and somehow it always felt that work came first, you know. She had papers at home all the time and I can remember her getting angry sometimes when I disturbed her. I guess she cared for me, she was working for the money to keep us and everything. But she seemed distant somehow.'

Martin nodded and responded, 'So, passed around, felt like you were everyone's problem, your mum got angry when you disturbed her but you think she worked because she cared.'

'Yeah, I'm sure she cared but I guess I didn't really feel it. And then when I was older, well, I didn't get to see as much of her as I wish I had, looking back. She died of a heart attack, it was so sudden, no real warning. She had never really stopped being active in her work, writing books and papers, you know, travelled around a fair bit too, to conferences. She was quite well respected in her field. Now I wonder sometimes how much I really got to know her. We had time together, weekends away, visits, time together doing ordinary things, but it always felt a bit rushed somehow. Either she had a deadline to meet or had to head off somewhere, or I had to get back to work.'

Mandy went quiet. She had realised something which somehow she felt she must have known, but suddenly now it was all too clear to her. She could feel herself go strangely cold and she could sense the frown spreading on to her face. 'Oh shit!' she exclaimed, and took a deep breath. And went quiet again.

Martin kind of sensed what Mandy had just recognised, but he wanted her to voice her sense of being like her mother in her own time and in her own way. He reflected her exclamation as a question, 'Oh shit?'

'I'm just like her, aren't I? I mean, being busy all the time. I'd never stopped and really thought about it like this before, it had always seemed the natural thing for me. I like being busy, that's how I am. It's only recently that I began to question it. I'm like my mother, and it killed her. Oh God.' The expression on her face had turned to one of shock and it seemed as though some of the colour had drained out of her cheeks.

'Quite a shock to think you may be like her in the way you keep busy with work,' Martin responded, pronouncing the words gently so as not to disrupt whatever Mandy was experiencing inside herself, yet ensuring that she knew he had heard what she had said and could experience hearing it for herself.

'It feels like the person I have been all these years, it's like not knowing who I am. But I know who I am at the same time. It's . . . it's so confusing.' Mandy could feel anxiety rising inside herself but she didn't quite understand why. She just knew that something was going on. She could feel herself trembling, as though she was cold, but she wasn't that cold. It was as though her nerves were on edge. She couldn't stop herself. She didn't understand what was happening. The anxiety was rising and she began gasping for breath, she found it hard to breathe out to take in the next breath. It was as though her lungs didn't want to work.

She's going into a panic attack, Martin realised, as he saw Mandy begin to tremble and start gasping for breath. 'Mandy, you're having an anxiety attack. Please listen to my voice if you can. You need to breathe slowly. Don't breathe in so deeply. And focus on my voice.' He was deliberately keeping his voice clear but calm. He needed to reassure her. 'It's OK, Mandy, it's OK. You have had a shock but it is going to be OK.' He could see how tense she was, her shoulders had risen and she was gripping the arms of the chair. 'Close your eyes and breathe slowly and rhythmically, and try to gently loosen your grip on the arms of the chair. Try and imagine the tension in your body dropping away, dropping to the floor.'

Mandy could hear what Martin was saying but it was difficult. God, was it difficult. She had never felt anything like this before. Her muscles felt so tight. Her breathing was relaxing a little now. She was able to breathe in again at will, and she swallowed on each out breath before breathing back in, each time through her mouth.

'Try and breathe in again through your nose, Mandy, and try and keep it to a steady rhythm. That's great, just keep with it. And try and let your shoulders drop a little, try and let their own weight drop them down a little.'

Mandy had got into a slow rhythm of breathing in through her nose and out through her mouth, slowly, slowly. Yes, she could feel the tension beginning to drop out of her arms and shoulders. Her chest still felt a little tight but not so much as it had been. She looked across at Martin and smiled weakly. Martin picked up the glass of water that was next to her and passed it to her. 'Here, drink this, but slowly, sip it. I can get some more if you need it.'

Mandy took the glass. Yes, it was cool and refreshing. The tension eased a little more and her breathing had returned to normal again. She felt exhausted, physically drained.

'What happened?'

'You had an anxiety attack, Mandy. I guess what was happening for you just now triggered it.' Martin was aware of a feeling of protectiveness for Mandy. She still looked shocked and somehow quite vulnerable. He decided not to push Mandy back towards exploring what had happened, she needed time to recover. To keep her where she was in the present, he asked, 'How are you feeling now?'

'A little better but very drained. It feels like someone has pulled out the plug and all my energy has flowed down the plughole. I feel glued into the chair, heavy, like a magnet is holding me here. Holding this glass up is taking an effort.'

'Take your time. Just relax for a bit. No need to say anything unless you want to.'

> Anxiety or panic attacks can be very frightening and debilitating, and they can occur within counselling sessions, particularly where something shocking or overwhelming occurs for the client. Here, Mandy has been shocked by her realisations that for all these years she has been just like her mother, and her mother had died. She may feel able to process it in the session, she may not. It is important from a person-centred perspective to trust the client to know what is right for her. The client will, however, be feeling very vulnerable.

'Thanks,' Mandy replied and blew out a deep breath. 'Thanks.' She lapsed back into silence. She wasn't really thinking, in fact, she felt quite blank. It was too much effort to think or even feel anything. She really felt like her energy had drained away. She felt like, what did she feel like? Yes, like an undercooked pancake that had been tossed and had landed in the chair. What an image, she thought to herself and realised she was smiling.

Martin had noticed the smile, and smiled back, aware that empathy can take the form of reflected body language as much as it can take the form of words.

Mandy felt she had to explain herself. 'I was just thinking about what I felt like and I had the image of a rather undercooked pancake being tossed in the air and landing on this seat in a "what the heck" kind of manner.' She blew out another breath. 'I hope that doesn't happen again.'

'You don't want to go through that again, yeah?'

'Too right.' Mandy paused. 'Will I? I mean, it's happened once. Thank God you were here, I mean, what if I'd been on my own. What if. ...' Her breathing began to get difficult again.

Martin noticed it. 'Take it easy, Mandy, you can control it, remember to keep your breathing light. Think of the pancake, how it must feel,' and he added to try and lighten it up for Mandy, 'all slopped on to the seat.'

Mandy had closed her eyes, and hearing the description of the pancake slopped on to the seat, felt herself smiling. She swallowed and got control of her breathing. She opened her eyes again. The tightness had eased pretty quickly, before it had got hold of her.

'I need some more water.'

Martin realised the glass was empty so he picked it up. 'I'll just fill it up from the water dispenser, OK for a minute?'

'Yes, I think so. Thanks.' She turned and looked out of the window. The tree caught her eye again. She breathed in deeply, closed her eyes and let her breath out. What a session this was turning out to be, she thought. I do need to think about what to do if this happens again. She decided not to dwell on it but wait until Martin returned. He came in and gave her the glass.

'Thanks.' She took a few sips. 'So, what do I do if it happens again?' Martin was aware that Mandy was asking him for direct advice and he knew it was respectful and empathic to her need to respond.

'Well, what we just did was what you need to do. What was most helpful just now?' Martin wanted Mandy to be able to affirm for herself what had been helpful so she could value it as a resource and begin to trust herself to cope.

It can be tempting to suggest that if a particular setting triggers her anxiety she should leave, but that could have the negative effect of reinforcing her anxiety. If it turned out that crowded or open spaces triggered the reaction, for instance, repeatedly leaving the environment could risk the onset of agoraphobia. Sometimes people can react in crowds, or in enclosed spaces, or in large superstores where they can feel overwhelmed by everything.

'Closing my eyes and hearing what you said about the pancake!' She smiled as she said it. 'That somehow helped me get control of my breathing.'

'OK, so something that affects you in such a way that it diverts your attention, and perhaps with a sense of the ridiculous about it.'

'Yes, I guess if I can blot out my surroundings for a few moments and try and do something to focus on something else.'

Martin had a suggestion he often made, and feedback from clients was that it could help. 'Why not carry a couple of photos around with you, one with a happy memory attached to it and the other of some humorous moment? You also need to cut down the oxygen supply so sometimes covering your face with a brown paper bag does the trick. Maybe try and think of being like a pancake again as well.' Martin added this in a kind of off-the-cuff way to try and get an amused reaction. It worked. Mandy burst out laughing. Martin was pleased as it would help to reinforce this reaction to the image.

'OK, I can go with that.' She was still smiling, but then her facial expression became more serious again. 'But I couldn't breathe out. I started thinking of my mother and her heart attack. I mean, it couldn't happen to me, like that, in that state, could it?'

Martin sought to reassure her. 'Highly unlikely, but if it would put your mind at rest, talk to your GP.' He was aware that he had stepped out of a counselling role, yet he sought to maintain the therapeutic attitudes of the person-centred approach. He needed to be authentically himself with Mandy, empathic to her concerns while offering warm acceptance of her as a person. 'I hear the anxiety in your voice, Mandy, it is a frightening experience.'

Clients do ask direct questions and they genuinely want a response rather than an opportunity to explore the question. Empathic sensitivity will enable the counsellor to draw a clear distinction if it is present. In this session, Martin has made suggestions regarding coping with an anxiety attack and has now been asked for his opinion concerning the client's risk of a heart attack. He has offered his ideas and suggestions. Is this appropriate for a person-centred counsellor? He may justify it on the grounds that his responses emerged from his feeling empathically present in this relationship with Mandy. Is he offering his advice from a place of genuine concern, or to assert some sense of being more knowledgeable than his client? It is difficult to justify withholding something that is genuinely felt to be helpful. Also, it is not very respectful to the client to come across as avoiding a direct question.

Yes, and I rather hope it doesn't happen again. I'm beginning to feel a little calmer now, thanks.'

'I'm sure you don't want to experience that again. We have a handout about panic attacks and how to handle them. Would you like a copy?'

'Yes, that would be good. Thanks.'

Martin reached over to his file and leafed through the plastic sleeves. He took one out and handed it to Mandy. He was aware that time was passing and it was coming to the end of the session. He had not forgotten what the GP had told him about the fostering, and he almost mentioned it but remembered Mandy had already disclosed this. He was glad he had caught himself from saying anything. Now his focus must be on helping Mandy get ready to leave and face the week ahead.

Clients can be left feeling extremely vulnerable as a result of counselling, particularly where deep memories or feelings surface, or they find themselves confronted by the kind of experience Mandy has had. The counsellor can check how the client is feeling and whether she feels she might need any further support during the week. In this instance, it might be helpful to ask if the client feels she might wish to consult her GP between sessions if she feels that would be helpful.

'Thanks. I'm worried about what might happen if it happens again. I'll try and remember what you have been saying today, and I'm sure that this will help. A week seems a long time.'

'Yeah, what do you think would help?' Martin felt it was in keeping with his non-directive approach to counselling to encourage Mandy to think through for herself what might be helpful rather than him coming up with ideas.

'I wonder if the GP could give me something, although saying that I feel reluctant to take tablets or something unless I really need to. I guess I want a kind of safety net, you know?'

'You want something that will be a bit of a safety net and I hear your reluctance to take anything for the sake of it, is that right?' Martin replied, wanting to hold her in this place still.

'Yeah. So, should I book an appointment to see the GP? Or can you ask her to give me something?'

Martin was aware that he was thinking about his response. He didn't want to undermine Mandy by giving the impression the GP would only listen to him, but he was aware that the GP probably ought to know that Mandy had had that anxiety attack, and that it would be helpful and probably in his client's interest for her to be made aware.

'I guess you could either book an appointment halfway through the week if you feel that would be helpful, or leave it and request an emergency appointment if there's a problem. I can let the GP know the situation so she is aware of what you might want to see her about. I can leave her a short note if you like.'

'That would be good. If the GP is aware I think I'll feel a little easier, and I can go away and think about what to do. Thanks again.' Mandy felt a little more relaxed. She just felt a little safer somehow knowing that her doctor would at least not be totally in the dark if she called for an appointment.

'Well, time is up. You have gone through a lot this session and again you'll probably want to give yourself some time to reflect on it all.'

'Yes, I know. But I think it has been useful even though it was disturbing as well. I guess I'll need to prepare myself to explore all of this a little more next time. Part of me feels encouraged by all this, it somehow feels as though I am getting real with myself, yet I know another part of me is frightened by it all and is leaving me unsettled.'

Martin smiled. 'Mixed feelings. Well we can focus on whatever you feel you want to bring into the session. It's your time. So I'll see you next week, same time, same day?'

'Yes, thanks.' Mandy got up and headed out through the door which Martin had opened for her. 'Bye.'

'Bye, see you next week.' Martin returned to his chair and sat down to take a few minutes to reflect on the session. It seemed that Mandy may have picked up a trait of being busy from witnessing her mother's behaviour, or was it a genetic predisposition? The old question of whether personality traits were nurture- or nature-based. Maybe being active was genetic, but the focus that she placed her busy-ness on was her work and that was where her mother had placed the emphasis. He took out the file and wrote his notes.

Notes should be relevant and reflective of content and not interpretations of process. They provide a brief record of what actually occurred. Notes should be locked away on surgery premises.

Client case notes

Client felt positive after the last session, as if a weight had been lifted. She began to focus on work issues and choices/options, recognising the pressure she felt under as well as her wish to return to work. Reflecting on this led her to recognise her tendency to be busy so much of the time paralleled her mother's style of working. This was a shock to her and she had an anxiety attack within the session. Discussed her needs in the coming week. Agreed that I should let her GP know she had the anxiety attack in case she needs to see her during the week.

Points for discussion/action

- How would you have handled being given information about a client after counselling had already begun?
- Does it make for a better counsellor if he has had experience of issues similar to those of his clients? What are the pros and cons of this?
- The client refers to not having been listened to by a man before. How well do you think Martin handled this situation as a male counsellor?
- Are you confident of sitting with a client who has an anxiety attack, and of what to do to help them?
- Was it therapeutically helpful for Martin to offer to write a note to the GP? What other situation can you think of in which you might need to make a decision on this?
- Critically evaluate Martin's responses in this session from the standpoint of his empathy for Mandy.
- Make your own clinical notes of this session.

SUPERVISION I

Martin was attending his fortnightly supervision session with Anne, whom he had worked with for a couple of years. She also had experience of working in primary healthcare as a counsellor and he had found her experience very helpful. He sensed that it was important to be supervised by someone who had a sense of the culture of working within a GP surgery. He always introduced new clients to her and he had decided to start this supervision session by talking about Mandy. He was aware that a great deal had happened in those first two sessions and he felt he needed time to reflect on it and to discover whether he was missing anything that Anne might pick up on.

'I want to talk a bit about a new client, Mandy, who attended for the first session the week before last.' Martin was in the habit of disclosing his client's first name. He felt it made it more real for him when he talked about them, more personal. He wanted to communicate to Anne what he felt, what he was experiencing in working in therapeutic relationship with his clients.

'OK, tell me about Mandy and your experience of being in therapeutic relationship with her.'

'It has only been two sessions so far, but they have been intense. There is a lot happening for this client and I feel I am still only learning about her. She was referred by her GP. She had lost her motivation for her work – she is a busy marketing executive – and had come to the surgery very tearful and just struggling to hold it together. The GP felt she needed time to talk things through and referred her on to me.'

'OK, that sounds straightforward.'

'Well, yes and no. You know what it is like, someone is referred for what appears to be a straightforward issue but once they begin to talk, deeper problems become apparent, and this is certainly the case with Mandy. During that first session she became extremely tearful. At the time I did not know why, she spoke of missing someone so much. She then explained she was referring to her mother, who died five years ago. She said that she hadn't really cried for her, that she had got a new job around that time and had put all her energy into that.' Martin could feel how he had begun to speak more softly and he wasn't sure why. Anne had picked up on it too.

'Your voice changed as you were speaking, Martin.'

'Yes, I noticed that too.' Martin paused, closing his eyes to be a little more in touch with what was present for him. Anne allowed him the time he needed and did not disturb his process. He started to speak, still with his eyes closed. 'I feel a strong affection for her, I think affection is the right word.' He opened his eyes and looked over towards Anne. 'What were you sensing from my voice change?'

'It did sound as though you were speaking about someone you had great affection for, but at the time there was something for me about respect and fragility. I'm not sure what that was about.' Anne had felt that, as Martin spoke, he was almost trying to not speak in a tone that would be harsh and somehow damaging. She added, 'but your sense was for great affection', wanting to keep the focus on Martin's experiencing.

'Yes, affection, and while I want to pick up on respect and fragility, I also want to stay with affection and get a grip on it. It is clearly something that I am experiencing that is relevant to the relationship with this client and I feel I need to get clear what it is about.'

'So, what is the affection you feel for Mandy all about.' Anne voiced it as a statement rather than as a question and left a silence for Martin to fill with his own process of reflection.

Martin sat and tried to sense the tone of this affection. He wanted to think about it, yet he also wanted to put his mind to one side and be with this sensed affection and see what it led to.

In supervision it can be invaluable to explore the feelings that arise in relationships with clients. They generally have significance. Here, Martin has identified a feeling, 'affection', but it is too broad and he feels he needs to gain clarity on what it actually is. Rather than think about it, he chooses to be with the feeling, to enter more fully into it. It is helpful for counsellors to be clear as to whether feelings that arise within them in the counselling work are rooted in their own past experiencing or have arisen spontaneously through the experience of the therapeutic relationship. It could be that Mandy reminds Martin of someone and it has triggered a remembering of old feelings associated with that person, or it could be something in particular about Mandy and what she means to him as a person in her own right. By becoming clear to himself on these matters, Martin will be able to enter into a more fully congruent state which will be important when he sees Mandy for her next session.

Martin imagined himself back with Mandy again as clearly as he could, reliving in his imagination the point at which she mentioned her mother, and how it was to sit opposite her as she wept openly and released the pain of missing her mother. He remembered how he had asked about touching her arm. Oh yes, he hadn't mentioned that to Anne.

'I can see her sitting in front of me weeping, and I ask if it would help if someone touched her arm. She took her hand from her face and reached out, and I
touched her arm for a while. It was a kind of instinctive response, but I needed
to reach out.'

Anne was listening intently and trying to be with her own reactions as well, in
case she picked something up from within her experiencing that would be relevant to what Martin was describing.

Counsellors can miss things and a role of the supervisor when working from a
person-centred perspective is to be open to her own experiencing and to distinguish elements that become present in herself that may have relevance.
In the moment of deeper contact, thoughts and feelings can pass through the
counsellor unnoticed, even very obvious perceptions can be missed. The
supervisor hopes to pick up on these, often they are not the result of logical
thought but take the form of a spontaneous presence. The supervisor's congruence enables her to identify these elements as they can stand out quite
sharply sometimes and she has a responsibility to voice these. Of course,
sometimes these elements may not be picked up by the supervisor, but may
then be picked up by the person who supervises her supervision practice.

Anne felt an instinctive sentence forming which was not driven by logical
thought, it just appeared and demanded to be voiced: 'Who were you reaching
out for, Martin?'

The room was suddenly quiet, Martin could feel his heart had begun to thump in
his chest. Oh-oh, he thought, something is going on here. The moment Anne
had finished her question Martin knew the answer. It came in a flash, a clear
image of a sentence had formed in his mind. He voiced it. 'She could have been
my daughter.' He could feel his eyes moisten and he drew in a deep breath, held
it momentarily and breathed out deeply through his mouth. He opened his eyes
and looked across at Anne. 'She could have been my daughter.' He tightened
his lips. 'That's the attraction. That's why I used the word affection. I reacted to
her as if she was my daughter.'

Anne was nodding slowly and reflected back, 'reacted as if she was my daughter. . . .'

Martin shook his head. 'I hadn't realised I had quite such strong feelings. Well, I'm
not sure how strong they are but I am aware that they are there. Well, this
sense of deep affection is there.' Martin rested his chin on his right hand, his
elbow on his knee, and looked towards the window. He shook his head again
and took another deep breath, more measured this time. 'OK, so I have this
sense of affection, but I need to think about why, and why Mandy in particular.
I have worked with female clients of her age without this reaction cutting in.'

'Why Mandy? Why the strong affection for Mandy?' Anne reflected the questions
that Martin seemed to be communicating to her.

'Well it isn't that she reminds me of a daughter, because I don't have one. We only had two sons. We wanted, well, I wanted a daughter, but it didn't happen. And then after our second son was born, well, we split up a few years after. But why am I reacting to Mandy?'

Anne left the question in the air, allowing Martin time to reflect further. Martin was frowning and she could see his intense struggle to make sense of it. But he couldn't. He shook his head. 'I must be missing something, but I don't know what.'

'OK,' Anne replied, 'let's consider what you know about Mandy and see if that triggers anything.'

'OK, I've mentioned her job and the stress she is under. She is 36, single. She was fostered out as a young child, her mother was a researcher and put her time into building a career and to earn money. Mandy's father had left when she was four.' Martin could feel himself going quiet again and sensed a strange coldness creeping over him. 'Oh shit! I've got it. It's so obvious. I missed it. Her father abandoned her, Anne, her father abandoned her. Leaving my wife, I kind of abandoned my sons. I guess I was trying to compensate in some way.' He thought for a moment. 'Or was I just responding as a human being to another person in pain? How do I tell? It makes sense that it may have been some kind of compensation.' Martin stopped and thought again while Anne reflected Martin's dilemma.

'Were you compensating for your own perceived act of abandonment, or simply responding as a fellow human being to someone in pain.'

Martin frowned suddenly. 'But I didn't know she had been abandoned by her father at that point. That only came out in the second counselling session. All I knew at the time was that she was hurting for her mother. But then maybe at some deeper level I did know, that maybe some deep hurt in her touched into hurt or guilt within me? Questions and no real answers.'

Anne smiled, 'We don't always get answers, Martin, you know that. Sometimes we simply struggle with our experiences and it is that struggle that is the work that needs to be done. It may be that you picked something up somehow, though I am sure there will be many different explanations for this, or you may have simply felt a surge of compassion for Mandy in her distress. But you used the word affection and this is nagging away at me, so I guess I'm bringing it back to you as I don't feel this has been resolved.'

'And I still have one of the words that you used in my mind – fragile. She did seem fragile and it does feel like affection. It doesn't feel more than that. I don't feel any sexual attraction here, or anything like that. But there is something in my heart that goes out to her.' Martin shook his head again.

'Maybe it is OK to feel affection for our clients, Martin? Maybe it is OK.'

'I'd like to be clearer as to why. I am beginning to think about the time and I have other things to say about Mandy, but then I don't want to . . . I was about to say *abandon* this theme and then I realised what word I was going to use. There is something running here about abandonment. Look, I'm seeing my therapist first thing next week, I think that's the place to take this. Otherwise I am not going to focus on what else happened with Mandy or my other clients. Is that OK?'

Anne thought for a moment. She could see the logic. She didn't feel as though Martin was seeking to avoid issues. Her experience of him was that he was open and took a professional view of his need to know himself and make sense of his experiences with clients. 'OK. Let me know where it leads to and obviously we'll need to keep this in mind in the future. While I feel OK about it, I also feel I need to ask whether you feel OK working with Mandy?'

Martin thought about it for a moment, 'Yes, I do. And somehow more so given what we have just been discussing. I mean, stopping working with her would be another abandonment, wouldn't it? And with no other counsellors at the surgery, well, it's not that I could even refer her to a colleague. No. I'll keep with her. I feel I am going to learn something through all of this and maybe that learning will impact on Mandy and be helpful.'

Anne was aware of still feeling disturbed, and it was around her lack of clarity about Martin's feelings for Mandy.

'What feelings are present for you when you are with Mandy?'

Martin immediately had the image of her crying, of her distress when she had talked of the loss of her mother, and he recalled those words he had used in the last session. 'I care about her.'

'You care about her.' Anne kept her response brief and waited. She could sense Martin was concentrating on himself and felt trusting that he was ready to explore this further.

'I do. And I like her. I experience her as a nice person, and if I hadn't been her therapist, and given different circumstances, I'd have probably wanted to have got to know her.' Martin could feel his heart thumping a little. 'I have got feelings for her, haven't I? Yeah, I like her. And I feel for her as well, that loss, and what happened to her as a child, and not really feeling her mother's care for her.'

'Mhmm. I think it important to be clear about this, yeah? You care about her, you like her.'

'I do. And I know my boundaries as well.' Martin could feel a shift in himself as he said this.

'Yes, I know you do. I guess I wanted to give you the opportunity to connect with what is present for you so you could be clear, and I could be clear as well.'

'Yes. I do care about her, I do want her to come through this and move on. I really did feel some compassion for her, and I so sensed her sadness.' Martin sat for a moment and thought. 'People really do not appreciate what we person-centred counsellors experience by trying to stay open to what is present for our clients, and our own reactions. I felt so drained after that session. They see counselling as a soft option, particularly person-centred. OK. It feels good to openly acknowledge these feelings.'

Anne felt more relaxed and realised that the lack of clarity had cleared for her. She trusted Martin's professionalism and did not feel a need to say more on the topic. 'OK, so there was something else you wanted to say?'

'In the next session Mandy had an anxiety attack, almost verging on a panic attack.'

Anne's eyes widened. 'How was it?' she asked, 'and how were you?' She felt concern for how Martin might have been affected by the experience.

'I was actually very calm, talked her down calmly, sought to reassure her, made some suggestions as to how she might handle it or minimise it if it happened again.'

'Do you think it will?'

'I'm not sure. It arose out of her making a connection concerning her mother and herself. Mandy has always been busy and involved in her career. It turns out that her mother was the same, and as I said, Mandy was fostered out so that her mother could pursue her career. She had contact with her mother. When she did finally move back in with her mother she remembers her being angry if she was disturbed when she brought work home.'

Anne nodded.

'Well, Mandy had not made the connection between her "busy-ness" and commitment to work, and her mother, who had the same trait. It was a tremendous shock for Mandy and triggered the attack. She went very pale and struggled to find her breath. It left her, I think, really unsure as to who she was. I mean, who she is. That recognition on top of her tears of grief for her mother the previous week, and feeling overwhelmed by work and the demands and stresses of it all, well, I guess everything was just too much. But she was very shocked about suddenly seeing her mother in the way she is. My sense was that it really and profoundly disturbed her primary sense of self, her identity if you like. It seemed to crumble away and she was left feeling shocked and very vulnerable.'

Anne was aware that her concern had now shifted towards Mandy. 'So, what happened? Was Mandy OK? Did she need to see her GP?'

She was wobbly and nearly went back into it again, but managed to come out of it and regain control. We talked about what would be helpful and I suggested she consider making an appointment to see the GP. She felt she wanted to go away and think about it. I offered to send the GP a note to let her know what had happened in case Mandy called. I was a bit hesitant in suggesting this because I didn't want to undermine Mandy, but I also felt the GP should be aware.'

'Did you put it in writing?'

'Yes, I sent the GP a short note and kept a copy for my file.'

'Do you think she'll go to the GP?'

'She was concerned and it wouldn't surprise me if she has another attack. It is so difficult. I don't want to over-react and alarm Mandy even more, you know? And I'm not sure what the GP would do anyway. She could prescribe something, but I know she is a GP who prefers not to prescribe if possible and that she is aware that while medication can support therapy, it can also limit it by inhibiting the client's range of emotional experiencing. She has often held back prescribing to allow counselling to try and help the person first, where she has felt this to be safe and appropriate.'

Counsellors working in primary healthcare settings need to have an appreciation of medications that are likely to be prescribed for conditions such as depression, anxiety, panic attacks, racing thoughts, etc. Often a chemical intervention has been tried before counselling and clients may still be on the medication. It is likely to affect mood and the counsellor needs to take this into account. This is particularly so where clients have been prescribed tranquillisers, for instance benzodiazepines, which tend to flatten mood or can take out the peaks and troughs of mood swings. This can have the effect of stabilisation but in terms of therapy can remove the client's sensitivity and ability to engage with and express feelings. It can therefore limit the scope of counselling interventions. In other instances, mood stabilisers can buy time for patients to begin talking through issues and problems without encountering the extreme mood swings that can put them at risk, perhaps of suicidal ideation, intent and action or other forms of self-harm.

Anne nodded. 'Seems like you have it in hand. It also seems as though there is a lot for six sessions.'

'Yes, I know. I have made it clear to Mandy that the counselling is limited and I will mention this again next time. I think that before I see you again in two weeks we will have discussed whether Mandy needs more therapeutic intervention and I expect I shall be discussing this with her GP. It really frustrates me. There just does not seem to be an appreciation that clients can need more than six sessions and we counsellors are not given the professional credibility to make decisions about the number of sessions we offer clients. Damn rationing, that's what it is.'

'It isn't like that everywhere, but I know it is where you work and I really hear and appreciate your frustration. I'm sure you'll discuss it with Mandy and represent her needs to the GP.'

Martin breathed out heavily. 'Yeah. In the meantime I will trust Mandy to bring to the sessions what she feels she needs or wants to address given the time frame we are working within. Let's stop at that, as I want to move on to another client.'

Points for discussion/action

- Do surgery counsellors need to be supervised by someone who has experience of working in that setting?
- Were there elements from the counselling sessions that were not voiced by Martin, but which perhaps should have been?
- Should Anne have encouraged Martin to spend longer focusing on and exploring the affection issue?

- Did you feel that Anne was communicating the core conditions, and can you give examples where this is the case?
- If you had been Martin, how do you think you would have been left feeling after discussing Mandy with Anne?
- Critically evaluate the supervision session.

SESSION 3

Mandy was running late and she knew she was going to struggle to get to the counselling session on time, but when she had phoned the surgery, the lunchtime 'we are closed' message meant she couldn't let them know. Oh well, she thought, I tried. She arrived in the end just a couple of minutes late, walking briskly from the car park. She felt breathless as she told the receptionist she was there to see the counsellor.

She had only just sat down in the waiting room when Martin came out.

'Hello, Mandy, come on through.'

'Thanks. Sorry I'm a bit late,' she said, aware that she must have sounded breathless.

'Sounds as though you have been rushing,' Martin replied with a smile.

'Yes, and I think I am a bit unfit. Maybe I should get some exercise. Actually that's something I have been thinking about.'

They had now entered the counselling room and were sitting down.

'Thinking about some exercise then,' Martin reflected back.

In some surgeries it is quite a long walk to the counselling room, and there can be a dilemma around whether or not to enter into conversation or find oneself walking along, sometimes one behind the other, in stony silence. In this instance, a conversation has been struck up and having arrived in the counselling room Martin has offered Mandy the opportunity to continue with the fitness theme that she has mentioned.

'Well, I've been doing a lot of thinking this last week, a lot. And I've had a lot of time to do it as well. I was shocked by last week, no doubt about that. It really left me with a lot of questions, and not very many answers. It wasn't just the anxiety attack that got to me, it was the strength of feeling that was associated with it and which persisted for some time afterwards.'

Mandy seemed to be in full flow. Martin did not want to interrupt her, so he purposely nodded when he had her eye contact and said 'mhmm'.

'I had so many feelings around and, well, it took me some time to kind of sort them out a bit. In fact, that evening I just felt generally pissed off with myself, you know, just ... oh, I don't know, but I just felt I had had enough of feeling fed up. Kind of fed up with being fed up, so I cheered myself up with a bottle of wine. I don't normally drink much, but I felt I needed it and, oh, I felt grim the next day. I'm not used to it. Anyway, I just felt irritated with myself, irritated that I could find myself doing things that, well, that my mother did. Well, not exactly doing what she did, but getting caught up in this kind of "got to be busy all the time" way of think and acting.'

Martin continued to nod, aware that Mandy still seemed to have a lot to say.

'I got angry at her for being like that and making me like that. And then I felt guilty for feeling that way. I mean, she didn't make me become so busy all the time, but she sure gave me a role model. And I went along with it, all these years, I went along with it.' Mandy began to shake her head as she looked at Martin. 'What am I like? What am I like?' The first time she emphasised the *what*, the second time she emphasised the *am*. She stopped speaking.

Martin thought for a moment. Long summary or brief reflection? He pondered, but he knew he didn't have much time. One of the challenges of counselling is to somehow make these decisions and often it feels as though a choice hasn't been made. His instinct was always towards brief responses. He didn't want to get into some kind of monologue of a reflection that left his client feeling as though she was in the audience. So he sought to be brief but catch and reflect back what he experienced as key points.

'So, a lot of thinking, fed up with yourself, had some wine because you were fed up with being fed up, got irritated with yourself, angry at your mother, guilty with yourself, wondering how you managed to copy your mother and now left with "what *am* I like?" He deliberately said it fairly quickly, reflecting Mandy's tempo of speech these last couple of minutes.

'Yeah, what am I like? Who am I? What am I? What do I want? How do I want to be? So many questions.' Mandy shook her head. 'So many questions.'

Martin reflected back, 'So many questions,' and allowed the silence that followed to remain present.

Mandy was aware of the questions. She opened her mouth, closed it, and then smiled a broad grin.

'Martin instinctively turned his head slightly and raised his eyebrows as if to say 'Yes, tell me about it.'

'I was about to say, and God does this sum me up, I was about to say, "I need to *do* something." Doing! I want to try something else for a change.'

'Part of you instinctively wants to focus on *doing* while another part wants to seek something else.'

The notion that we contain within ourselves different urges or aspects of our nature is not uncommon. Yet it can prove valuable within a therapeutic dialogue for a client to begin to separate out the different aspects of themselves. These may be associated with particular thoughts, feelings or behaviours, and usually a combination of all three. The 'doing' aspect of Mandy has been a major driving force for many years, and it will have given her associated thoughts and feelings, probably all positive, which is why she has maintained this. Yet now she wants to cultivate a fresh way of being, though she has not yet defined exactly what this is. She wants another way and has begun the process of groping towards it, even though she is unclear as to what it is and how it will satisfy her.

'It feels like that, as if I am being pulled in different directions. I naturally want to do, keep busy, keep active, take the pressure. I thrive on it.'

'You thrive on pressure,' Martin reflected, knowing that either the part of Mandy that did just that would respond, or maybe the other part that didn't might emerge a little more strongly.

'Yes, I do. Well, I did.' Mandy paused. 'No, I do. It is part of who I am.'

'Part of who you are.' Martin had noted the shift. It was now only part, not the whole person driving onwards to more and more busy-ness.

'Yes, part of who I am.' Mandy stopped to think again. After a minute of silence, which Martin sensed to have been a working silence so he had not interrupted it in any way, Mandy continued. 'Yes, that's it. Part of who I am. But not all of who I am. I'm more than "busy me", aren't I?' She looked towards Martin, wanting an affirmation that this was so.

Martin registered this but did not want Mandy to gain affirmation from him, but rather he wanted her to trust her own experiencing in this moment. 'Sounds as though *you* are recognising that you are more than "busy me".'

'I am. I know I am, at least, I think I am.' Mandy could feel her sense of 'I am more than my busy me' sliding away a little. 'I must be, mustn't I?'

Again, Martin could feel the draw to make the affirmation for Mandy, but he did not want to do that just yet. He wanted her to have every chance to affirm it for herself. He recognised the importance of allowing her to develop an 'internal locus of evaluation'. Martin was suddenly aware that his thoughts had drifted and he had been wondering what Mandy was feeling about this idea of being more than her 'busy me'. He was not sure how long he had been lost in this train of thought, but he sensed a shift and Mandy was looking at him differently. She must have guessed I drifted away, and I need to own it, be authentic here. Maybe it is relevant.

'I drifted into my own train of thought there, wondering what you felt about the idea of being more than "busy me".'

'I'm not sure, really not sure. Seems to be lots of feelings, and they are, well, a bit muddled really. I mean, I kind of feel excited at the idea but really close to that feeling there is a concern as well. It feels kind of alien somehow. But I'm not sure what it is that feels so strange because . . . well, because I don't know what it is. I mean, sitting here, now, my mind is busy. I'm thinking, generating thoughts. I'm trying to make sense of it all, and it's making me busy. I don't want to be busy. I want to stop. I want to. . . I want to. . . ,' Mandy spoke with such passion, then lapsed into silence.

'You want to. . . ?' Martin replied, reflecting and holding Mandy on what she had just said.

'I want to just *be*.'

'You want to just *be*?' Martin reflected back.

'Yeah. I want to. . . ,' Mandy looked Martin in the eye. 'This'll sound weird. I want to be me. But I don't know who *me* is. At least I know who part of me has been but I don't know if that is the real me or a me that I picked up from my mother.'

Martin felt it was time to reflect back and give Mandy a chance to listen to what she had just said. He spoke slowly and deliberately so she had time to listen and absorb what she had been saying. 'I want to be me, but you don't know who that me is. You don't know if it is the real me or some me you learned from your mother.'

'Yes. I don't know who the real me is.' Mandy went silent again. She was thinking hard and yet she was not getting answers. Who is me? The thought kept ringing in her head. Who *is* me? No answer came. 'I don't know where to start. I mean, who am I? How do I find out? I don't want to carry on the way I have been. I know it has been good to me, you know, I have achieved a lot. But. . . . Yet it is all that I know. I don't know how to stop. I don't know how to stop.' Mandy burst into tears and hid her head in her hands. She sobbed and began to rub her eyes. Martin handed her a tissue. She took it gratefully. 'I feel like I'm going mad, Martin, I really do.'

First time she has called me by my name, Martin thought. He avoided making assumptions around this. He was aware that the room felt silent, as though there was some deeper connection present between them. He nodded slightly and replied, 'I'm sure it must do, Mandy.'

'I'm not though, am I?'

'No.'

There are times when it is right to help a client come to her own conclusions, and there are times when reassurance needs to be given. In this instance, Martin has judged it to be right to offer reassurance to Mandy. Some might argue that he is rescuing her from the sense of going mad. Maybe he is. Sometimes rescuing is a means of conveying a warmth and unconditional positive regard. Often with rescuing, the rescuer needs to ask if he is actually seeking to rescue the client, or himself, from engaging in difficult or uncomfortable feelings or thoughts.

'No. I'm sure I'm not. But I feel as though I am staring at some strange, new world, as though it has different rules or laws and I don't know what they are,

or how to be in that world. I feel...,' Mandy swallowed, 'I feel very alone.'
A short silence followed. Martin reflected back what Mandy had said.

'Facing a strange, new world, feeling very alone.'

Tears formed in Mandy's eyes again. She looked at Martin who could feel a shift in
perspective. Mandy somehow seemed to be moving away from him in some
strange way, and he was aware of a strange quiet in the room. He had experienced this before and it was often associated with connection to very deep feelings. It could feel unnerving but he knew he must stay with it and with Mandy.
Somehow this moment seemed hugely important, but he could not explain
why. He could see the tears rolling slowly down Mandy's face. She somehow
looked much younger, almost child-like. He sensed that she was feeling something powerful within herself and probably from her past.

He spoke gently. 'What are you feeling, Mandy?'

'Please don't make me.'

Martin was feeling extremely focused now and very, very aware that Mandy
might be about to disclose something highly significant. The thought of sexual
abuse crossed his mind but he let it pass.

'Please don't make you?' he responded, gently, quietly, not wanting to in any way
jolt Mandy out of her experience.

'Don't make me go. Please don't make me go. *Please*.' Mandy's voice was higher,
shriller, like a little girl who was desperate to try and stop something happening.

Mandy had reconnected with something deep in herself and seemed to be reliving
some event. He didn't know what it was. He didn't want to disturb her, but he
wanted to help her describe what was happening.

'Who's making Mandy go where she doesn't want to go?' was his response,
spoken softly and with as much warmth and gentleness as he could muster.
He could feel his spatial awareness shifting again.

'Please, mummy, please. I don't want to go. I want to stay here with you. Please.
Let me be with you. Please.'

Goosebumps broke out all over Martin's arms, the back of his neck and his scalp.
It's the fostering. I think she's reliving being made to go away. He instinctively
knew it was a time of great sensitivity and vulnerability for Mandy.

'Mandy doesn't want to go, does she?' he again spoke softly. He could feel his
own eyes beginning to water as well and a lump appeared in his throat.
He knew he was desperate to keep his voice steady. He mustn't get this
wrong. He knew he was feeling connected to Mandy and he had to stay with
that connection. He knew he could trust himself to say what was helpful if he
could keep that connection.

'No, she doesn't.'

Shit, thought Martin, she's gone into third person.

'Where don't you want to go, Mandy?' he asked, trying to bring her focus back
into herself as a child.

'Mr and Mrs Sharp.' Mandy was almost pouting now as she said this. Her face was
an image of sadness. But he must not say that, he did not want to instil anything into Mandy in this vulnerable and impressionable state.

'Mr and Mrs Sharp?' he reflected gently but questioningly.

'I have to go and live with them. I don't want to. I want to be with my mummy. I'm scared. Don't make me go, please don't make me go.'

'I'm not going to make you go.' Martin sought to reassure Mandy.

Mandy breathed in deeply and back out again. She was pouting and tears were still trickling down her face. She blinked twice and as she did so Martin could feel a change. He could not easily describe it but it was as though both he and Mandy had moved away from the encounter that had just happened. Things kind of felt solid again, somehow. He blinked as well and swallowed. Mandy took a deep breath and closed her eyes. 'What happened?' she asked.

'Were you aware of yourself just then?'

'Yes, I was, but I was powerless. It was like watching something happening, but it was happening inside me.'

'Can you tell me what you experienced?' Martin wanted to help Mandy engage with her experience and make her own sense of it.

'It was me when I was four years old, when I was being made to go, to be taken to Mr and Mrs Sharp. They were my foster parents. Well, they were actually distant cousins, but I think of it as being fostered. I didn't want to go. I pleaded not to go. My mother said I had to and that I had to be very brave. I didn't want to be brave. I wanted to be with my mummy. I loved her. I hated her too. I hated myself. I didn't settle down with them for a long while.' Mandy was speaking in an almost disconnected kind of way. Each sentence was followed by a short silence. She looked kind of vague as she spoke. 'I did still see my mother. Not as much as I wanted. I missed her. I loved her. I hated being there. Well, at first anyway. I did get to like it. I guess I got used to it. I blamed them. I blamed myself. They had me for nearly three years. While my mother established her career. She worked away. I saw her some weekends. I got used to it. Mr and Mrs Sharp were very kind. They are both dead now. They were quite old even then. Well they were to me. I think they were in their fifties. They had never had children of their own. I suppose it had seemed like a perfect solution.' Mandy stopped speaking.

Martin had a sense that Mandy was still partly in her four-year-old experience and partly in the present. He was aware that he couldn't hurry this. 'A long time ago yet it must feel so real.'

'Yes.' Mandy could feel herself stuck in this strange state. She was aware of what she had been saying but it seemed to be coming out without her having any real conscious involvement in the matter. It wasn't a very pleasant experience and she wanted to come out of it. She closed her eyes and tried to collect her thoughts. She felt very sweaty. She forced herself to yawn to try and bring herself out of it. It helped, but her head still felt as though it was full of a warm fog made from droplets of treacle. She blinked heavily a few times and yawned again. She became aware of how tight her back felt. She stretched. That helped. She felt she was coming back into her self. She took a slow, deep breath, held it and breathed out slowly.

'I think I'm back. That was some experience. I could hear myself speaking but I somehow didn't feel ... didn't feel kind of. . . .' Mandy paused. 'This will sound daft but I somehow didn't feel me, no, I mean I didn't feel. . . . It's hard to describe. I was disconnected somehow from myself, like I was not quite where I should be.' She shook her head. 'But I heard every word. I felt every word too. I haven't thought about any of this in years. But it seemed so vivid, so real. It's all part of me, isn't it?'

Mandy could feel herself in a very reflecting state all of a sudden. She didn't feel like she really wanted to say anything. She felt she wanted to just sit quietly. 'I just want to sit quietly. I'm not sure that I want to explore anything more just at the moment. I just want to sit quietly. I feel as though I have been pulled apart and am coming back into myself again, but I'm different, and I can't define what it is that's different, but it's different. I feel calmer, relaxed, almost. . . .' Mandy hesitated. 'Almost at peace in some way that I can't explain. I want to just sit with it. Do you mind?'

'No. Not at all. Can I get you anything?'

'No. Actually, yes, a glass of water. My mouth is incredibly dry.'

Martin went off to get the water and Mandy sat. She was aware that one moment she was aware of thinking and the next she was just sitting without any thoughts in her head. I'm doing nothing, she suddenly realised. I'm just sitting and *being* and it's OK.

Mandy may have entered into a dissociated state, the traumatised aspect of her structure of self reflected through the four-year-old that had been so deeply affected by being taken away to live with the Sharps. She had been aware of what she had been saying, but had felt powerless to stop it, as though this part of herself had taken her over. It is a not uncommon experience for clients who have experienced profoundly shocking trauma. It leaves the client in a vulnerable state and particular care is required when working with people in this condition.

Much work has been done on this area of work from a person-centred perspective in terms of 'fragile process' and 'dissociated states' (Warner, 1991, 1998, 2000). There can be more than one dissociated state and the challenge for the counsellor is to be attentive to all aspects of the person, allowing each to feel warmly accepted and listened to as the client moves between them. In this instance, Mandy's four-year-old state has emerged along with the feelings associated with being made to go and live away from her mother. These feelings had previously been submerged, Mandy being unaware of them. Now they have become recognised and experienced by her, offering the possibility of healing.

Martin came back with the glass of water. She sipped it gratefully.

'Thanks. I was just sitting here and became aware that I was doing nothing, just sitting, just being here without any sense of urgency or need to do anything. I am just being, and it feels strangely satisfying.' She shook her head. 'Do all your clients experience this kind of thing?'

'Some do, some don't. Everyone's an individual with their own needs, their own process.'

'Yes, I guess so.' Mandy took more sips of water. 'I think I need to get up and move around a bit. I need to get myself more into my body and feel the floor.' She stood up and walked around, pressing each foot down on to the floor with deliberation. 'That's better. I think I'm getting ready to feel able to face the world again.'

Mandy sat down. 'You know, I can't carry on with my work any more. I have to do something different. I will have to go back, I can't afford to just stop, but I will have to do something else. Something. . . ,' she thought about it for a few moments. 'Something simpler.'

'Something simpler sounds good to you, huh?' Martin replied, seeking to reflect not just the words but the spirit of what Mandy had said.

'Yes, something simpler. Something has shifted in me and I don't know what it is. But I know I feel different and I know I have to act on this feeling, consolidate it in some way. It's precious, I don't want to lose it.'

Martin nodded. 'Seems like you have found something really precious, really important, something of great value.'

'Yeah, something I've never had before. It feels so. . . ,' Mandy looked surprised. 'This will sound odd, it feels very powerful but this is a different kind of power to what I have felt before. I'm used to power being very active and dynamic, but this feels measured, steady somehow. Yet I also still feel a little bit kind of out of phase with the world. Like part of me is still slightly out of sync.' She smiled, 'But it feels good even though it is a little weird.'

Martin nodded. 'I'm wondering what you want to do with the rest of the time we have today. There's still about 20 minutes of the session left.'

'I don't feel I can do any more. I feel emotionally, physically and mentally quite drained. I actually feel as though I want to go to sleep. Do you mind if I head off? I don't want to stop coming, but I really don't feel I can cope with any more today. It has been very powerful and it has made me realise how much I am affected by my past. It still lives on within me. But I also know that I do not have to sort of keep reliving it. I can move on. I have to move on. But I'm not sure quite what that means yet. I know it means change, inside and out. But I don't feel I want to start thinking about that now. I think I just need to rest and absorb what I have experienced today.'

'Sure you feel up to heading off? Do you want to sit a little longer?' Martin was concerned and wanted to communicate that to Mandy.

'No, I feel I'm coming back to being me again. I'm not going to drive off straight away. I will have a short walk and then come back for the car. I may get a coffee at the café over the road. I'll be fine. I just need some time to be with myself. Sounds funny saying that, but that's what I feel.'

'OK. Same time next Thursday?'

'Yes please. I'm not sure what I'll want to talk about. I need to let all this settle down first. I hadn't expected any of this today. I was planning to talk about my options for work and for making changes in my life generally. Still, maybe this will help me become a little clearer as to what I do and don't want. I guess time will tell.'

'I guess it will,' was Martin's response. He smiled and got up to open the door. Mandy turned as she walked through the door and reached out and shook his hand. 'Thanks. I'm not yet quite sure what I'm thanking you for, but it feels like I'm heading in the right direction here.'

Martin smiled and replied, 'I'm sure you are. Take care of yourself and I'll see you next week.' He watched Mandy head back down the corridor towards the waiting room and the exit. He took a deep breath. He hadn't really thought about how it had left him feeling. He felt incredibly tired and his head was heavy. He realised he needed some fresh air before writing his notes. He went outside for a walk around the surgery and sat for a while on the seat at the back. The air was cool and the breeze brought a welcome relief. He realised how hot he had become during that encounter. It had been intense. He wasn't sure quite what Mandy would make of it, but he trusted her process. What had happened he was sure was a necessary part of her healing process. It had not been forced. It had arisen spontaneously in response to . . . , what was it? Oh, yes, feeling very alone, facing a strange new world. That's what she had said. My God, he thought, what do we all carry around with us? What a struggle it is to liberate ourselves from negative conditioning and from memories and patterns that get so ingrained. Yet he recognised, too, that Mandy really was using the sessions. This wasn't a client who came in and didn't know what to talk about (as was sometimes the case). It seems she had come along at just the right time. Maybe that's the secret, he thought, the right timing. You can't force it. But you can sure get in the way of it! Mandy had come along at a point in her life when she was ready for change, although at the start she was not aware of it in those terms. The lack of motivation was merely a symptom. Now she was facing that strange new world, feeling alone, but seemingly prepared to go for it. It felt good to be part of Mandy's process of change, to feel that he was contributing to growth and perhaps her finding or even realising newer, certainly fresher, and perhaps even fuller potential within herself. He got up and went back in to write his notes.

Client case notes

Client began by experiencing her 'busy me' sense of self and recognised that she is made up of different parts. She recognised how difficult it felt to think about changing from 'busy me'. Client then engaged with feelings and experiences associated with her four-year-old self linked to being fostered. While she loved her mother as a child, she hated her foster parents (at first) and blamed herself. It was a lonely experience and was triggered into her awareness by feeling alone facing change in her present-day life. The experience left her feeling calmer, stronger and somehow more ready to face making changes. She mentioned feeling that she could not continue with her current job.

Points for discussion/action

- Was it appropriate for Martin to continue with the theme introduced in conversation outside of the counselling room?

- At what point does therapeutic relationship begin in such a situation?
- Discuss the associated thoughts, feelings and behaviours that could be associated with a 'busy me' sense of self or, as has more recently been described, in terms of 'configurations within self' (Mearns and Thorne, 2000).
- What is your theoretical explanation, from a person-centred perspective, of Mandy's reconnection with her experiences as a four-year-old.
- Critically evaluate Martin's responses in this session from the standpoint of his unconditional positive regard for Mandy.
- Make your own clinical notes of this session.

SESSION 4

Martin really did not know what to expect from the next counselling session with Mandy. He always sought to not anticipate, believing that it was important to be open to what clients brought with them. He did not plan anything himself, this being a hallmark of the person-centred approach. His intention was to listen to his clients and convey his empathy for what they were communicating as accurately as he could, offer them warm acceptance for the person that they are and to be authentically himself. He wanted to be open and spontaneous so that the dialogue between his client and himself flowed naturally. He did not wish to direct his client towards any particular focus. He had noted already with Mandy how themes emerged, how feelings surfaced without his having to in any way force the process.

So far each session had been intense and he wondered how Mandy coped between sessions. It was tempting to think back over the sessions that they had as he prepared to see her today, but he resisted this, preferring instead to be with himself quietly, seeking to be in touch with his own experiencing in readiness to receive Mandy into the counselling room. He trusted that what would emerge within the therapeutic climate he created with her would be pertinent. Mandy knew there were only six sessions and he trusted that she would have thought about this and would bring to the session what she wanted to deal with. He was also aware that her own structure of self, containing, as it did, elements that she might be unaware of, would also be making its presence felt, and hopefully more fully than she usually experienced.

By offering the attitudinal values of the PCA, the counsellor is creating an environment that encourages the client to grow towards a fuller and more accurate experience of herself. The client is likely to learn to trust her own inner prompting, if you like her own inner wisdom, as she seeks to make choices. Thoughts and feelings have emerged for Mandy in the previous sessions, causing her to engage more fully with aspects of her nature that were previously less to the fore. The therapeutic conditions will have provided a safe atmosphere for her, encouraging her to risk being more fully herself, even when that means different aspects of herself emerging that can feel quite distinctive from her everyday experiencing.

The receptionist knocked on the door, jolting Martin away from his reflection. 'Your first client has arrived, Martin.'

'Thanks,' he replied, 'I'll come out to her.' Martin got up and walked down to the waiting room. He noticed that Mandy was sitting wearing much more informal clothes, jeans and a shirt. It made him realise how formally she had been dressed before, dressed perhaps more in her work clothes. Interesting, he thought, I wonder what that is about? Maybe she is feeling more relaxed. He noted the question and put it to the back of his mind. He didn't plan to raise it unless it arose within the session in the context of whatever was being explored.

'Hello, Mandy, would you like to come through?'

'Thanks.' They entered the counselling room and sat down.

'So,' Martin began, 'how do you want to use this session?'

'Whenever I leave here I seem to have so much more to think about, so much to try and make sense of. I was really surprised by what happened last week. I did not expect to experience what I did. But I am glad that it happened. I can really grasp that I carry within me a sense of myself as a four-year-old. It left me thinking about how I live that out, and I realise that there is a part of me, quite a strong part, that doesn't like to be made to do things, or be told to do something that I don't want to do. And it can be very strong, to the point of being bloody-minded. I can see now where I get that from.'

'So your sense of being bloody-minded you can see links back to that four-year-old part of you.' Martin kept his empathic reflection simple and focused on the conclusion Mandy had presented, allowing her the opportunity to develop her theme further.

'Yes, and I can see that at times it is a strength, but at other times it can get in the way.'

'Get in the way?' Martin asked, and promptly realised that he had probably directed her away from a focus on it as a strength. Mandy responded before he had a chance to add anything else.

'Yes, when I feel pushed I think I stop listening. I put a kind of barrier up. I don't want to know. I become focused entirely on not giving way, not giving ground to whoever or whatever is pushing me. And I'm sure that is linked back to that early experience when I had to give way, when I had no choice in the matter.'

'So your sense is that when you are pushed you stop listening and become focused on not giving ground. A barrier comes up, yeah?'

Mandy nodded. 'And it's a very strong barrier, heavy, like a kind of, well, rather like a steel shutter.'

'Mhmm, like a steel shutter.' Martin was aware that as he said this he could really sense this image of a steel shutter slamming down hard with a loud clank.

'It's very thick and heavy, it blots out sound, hence I stop listening.'

'Thick, heavy, blotting out the sound, stopping you listen.' Martin nodded gently as he reflected back what Mandy had said.

'It feels kind of protective. I'm quite small and vulnerable behind it. I don't want to be small and vulnerable any more. I want to be strong like the shutter. That sounds crazy because in a way I am that shutter, but I'm not in control of it.

I want to feel it is part of me that I can choose to bring down when I want to. At the moment I react. I don't want to react. I want to...,' Mandy thought for a moment.

Martin remained quiet, allowing her this quiet thinking time, and wanting her to be sure of formulating in her own words exactly what it was that she wanted to be. He wanted her to listen to herself and express whatever thoughts or feelings arose in her, as he recognised that whatever it was going to be, it would be something that in voicing she would feel a sense of satisfaction towards.

'I want to stop reacting and be in command of my response,' she said finally, and looked very pleased with what she had said. She looked stronger somehow for having said it. Martin was curious as to what she actually meant.

'You want to stop reacting and be in command of your response.' He spoke slowly but with a tone of affirmation in his voice, allowing the words to have their impact on Mandy.

'Yes, I want to be able to choose how to be. I don't want to feel driven by history. I want to be able to hear what is being said, think it through, be aware of my feelings and respond in a manner that reflects my experience. I don't want to be pushed around, but I want to be clear in myself when I respond. I think I am like this, but not when I'm pushed. I can see this now. I need to realise that I am not four years old, that I am a woman with my own power.' Mandy emphasised the word power. She brought her hand up and covered her mouth. 'Can I?' she said, in a quieter tone.

Martin had noted her hand movement. 'I hear you affirming yourself as a woman with power, and I noticed you do this.' As he finished his sentence he lifted his own hand to his mouth in the same manner as had Mandy. 'And I heard a doubt in the way you said "can I?".' Martin had the feeling that this gesture was a bit like a little girl who has just said something she thinks she shouldn't have said, and covers her mouth instinctively. He didn't voice this, he didn't want to project an interpretation on the gesture.

'It was instinctive,' Mandy replied. She had already taken her hand away, but now she put it back in front of her mouth.

'Mhmm,' Martin nodded slightly, 'instinctive.'

'Yes, like I felt that I'd said something that I shouldn't have said.' Mandy felt herself feeling smaller as she said this.

'Something you shouldn't have said?' Martin responded with a hint of questioning in his voice.

'I am a woman with my own power.' Mandy stopped and thought for a moment. This time she had not raised her hand. She repeated it, emphasising the 'I', '*I* am a woman with my own power.' She smiled. 'That felt good. I want to say it again.'

Martin nodded and lifted and opened his hands to acknowledge that it was her space. He chose not to say OK as he didn't want to sound as if he was giving her permission. He wanted her to claim the moment and fill it with what she needed to do.

Mandy repeated her affirmation, this time the emphasis came out on the 'am'. 'I *am* a woman with my own power.' And again, shifting the emphasis once more.

'I am a woman with *my own power*.' She went silent, and her head bowed. Martin sensed that something unexpected had happened for her. Somehow she didn't seem so powerful. He decided to let her know that he sensed something had happened but he did not want to make any assumptions.

'What's happening for you, Mandy?' She remained silent.

The silence continued for a minute or so. Finally Mandy looked up and met Martin's eye contact. 'This is so silly, but it feels enormous.' Her hand had gone back over her mouth again. 'I'm feeling blocked. I want to say....' She shook her head. 'I want to say....' She shook her head again. 'I can't say it. I have to say it. This is ridiculous.'

'You want to say, you have to say...,' Martin replied, trying to hold the focus on the urge to say something that Mandy was struggling with.

Mandy heard Martin, and she drew her lips together and tightened them. She spoke softly, Martin had to really listen to hear the words Mandy was saying. 'I am a woman. . . .' She was quiet again.

Martin heard what Mandy had said and he felt unsure what to say.

Should he reflect it back in some way, or leave it and allow Mandy to say or do what she felt she needed to do without his interference. He was aware of not knowing what to say. As a man he felt strangely odd contemplating saying, 'I am a woman', a straight reflection. But he didn't feel at ease with saying 'you are a woman' either. Dammit, he thought, if I *was* a woman I wouldn't have this dilemma.

Once a person-centred counsellor is losing himself in thinking about a response to a client, then there is an issue or something that is getting in the way. The longer it goes on, the more distant the counsellor becomes from the client's frame of reference. If the counsellor can note that he is not responding and that there is a block, and put it aside, then he can regain connection with the client. If the block persists it may have relevance to the therapeutic relationship and need voicing. Either way, it is likely to be an issue to discuss in supervision.

The silence continued.

Mandy was lost in her own struggle. She was quite unaware of Martin. She was feeling utterly stuck. She knew she was a woman, of course she was, but somehow she was finding it so hard to say those four words. Her eyes were closed, her hand was against her mouth. She ran them through her head again and again, switching the emphasis as she did so. *I am a woman. I am a woman. I am a woman. I am a woman.* She was aware of moving her lips as she thought the words. *I am a woman.* 'I am a woman.' She realised that the words had come out audibly. She looked up.

'You are a woman.' The words came out of Martin's mouth completely involuntarily, and they felt right to say. A thought ran through his head, this feels like a four-year-old giving birth to an adult.

'Yes, I am a woman, and I have my own power. I have my own power.' Mandy
was speaking slowly and deliberately. She swallowed and nodded her head. She
was aware that she was gazing into space, not really thinking anything, just
sitting. 'I don't think I've ever felt like this before.'

Martin frowned slightly, he was not sure what Mandy meant. 'Haven't felt like
what before?'

'I feel different. I feel somehow more adult.' She paused. 'I feel like a woman and it
feels strange.'

'Feels strange feeling like an adult, feeling like a woman,' Martin reflected back.

Yes, strange and yet,' Mandy paused again, 'and yet normal as well. I feel calm, I
feel good. I feel strong.'

Martin just nodded, allowing Mandy to be with what she was experiencing while
seeking to communicate his attention to her.

'I do feel strong.' She smiled. 'I am a woman and I have my own power.' Mandy
breathed in deeply. 'Yes,' she said as she breathed out. 'Yes.'

'A strong and powerful woman,' Martin responded, speaking slowly and affirma-
tively.

'Yes I am, and now I have to figure out how to use this power. It's very energising.' She bit her lip and stared ahead of her. 'I have to make some changes to my
life, some radical changes. But I'm not going to rush anything. I don't want to
be reactive. I want to think it through and explore my options. I want to know
what choices I have, and then I want to weigh them all up and make decisions,
decisions for me.' Mandy paused before continuing. 'I feel like I'm waking up,
Martin, I feel like I'm waking up.'

'Waking up and wanting to make decisions for you,' was Martin's response.

Mandy nodded. 'Decisions for me, thought-through decisions. OK.' Mandy took a
sip of water. 'OK. I want to spend some time looking at my options. I know I've
got to get back to work and I know we have only got two more sessions. I want
to make the most of them. I feel I've really benefited from this, but I need to look
at some practical things. I want to use some time to look at my work in terms of
what it is giving me and whether I still want this. And if not, what do I want?
Can we do this?' She looked at Martin.

'We can use the time however you want to use it.'

Martin was struck by the apparent suddenness of Mandy's switch to a focus on practical needs. He realised that he was still thinking about what had just been happening and realised he had to make a quick adjustment. He had been thinking about Mandy claiming her womanhood, and wondered what that meant to her. But this was his wondering. Mandy seemed quite clear that she wanted to shift the focus of the session, and he wished to honour that. He wanted to be centred on his client's needs. He didn't feel unduly concerned at the shift, he had simply noticed that he had lagged behind a bit. He wondered whether that was significant in any way, and made a mental note to discuss it in supervision. He was aware that it had been an intense period and he felt it would be helpful to talk through his experience of what had happened, particularly so as he was a man, albeit almost old enough to be Mandy's father. That was a dynamic he hadn't thought about before. Maybe he ought to explore that in supervision. He didn't have a daughter, though, as he had mentioned to Anne. He made a mental note to reflect on this after the session. He recognised how easy it could be to respond from a particular identity within his own structure of self and he wanted to be clear that he was being present as Martin the counsellor and not Martin the father.

'OK. I really want to begin by looking at what my job gives me and what I would lose if I gave it up. Somehow, since that experience just now, I feel much more detached from work. It somehow doesn't feel quite so important.' Mandy was aware of feeling quite detached from thinking about work. It didn't stand out. Work felt somehow distant.

'Work doesn't feel so important,' Martin reflected back.

'No, at least, well, I mean, I know it is important but it somehow doesn't feel so pressing somehow.'

Martin had noticed the way Mandy had stumbled a bit over her words and also seemed to be indicating a split between what she was thinking and what she was feeling.

'Seems to me from what you have just said that you know it is important but your feelings are giving you another experience. Feels to me like a kind of split.' Martin was wanting to express his sense of what he had heard from Mandy's description of her experience.

'Yes, it does feel like a split. It is as though my head is saying one thing but my heart is saying something else. I know work is important, I need to work and I know that I get a lot out of it. I know I'm good at it, I've been successful and I like that. It gives me a good feeling. But I have other feelings as well, and these I guess are kind of new. I somehow don't feel connected with work.' Mandy paused momentarily to think. 'Maybe that's partly because of being off work, but I don't feel that it is just that. It feels much more like I have shifted inside myself. I don't feel comfortable at the thought of going back to work in the same way as I have in the past. I know I can't do that. It seems sort of clear and confusing at the same time. Am I making any sense?'

Martin wondered which aspect of what Mandy had just said to respond to. 'Seems like you are not sure whether it is making sense to you. Head says one thing, heart says something else.'

Martin deliberately did not go into detail with his empathic response, hoping that by keeping his response general Mandy might elaborate a little more and perhaps connect more deeply with her thoughts and her feelings. He was also conscious of not wanting to direct her to either her thoughts or feelings, but leave it open for Mandy to focus on that area of herself that she felt she needed to. The PCA does not encourage counsellors to be experts on their clients, and to think they know what is best for them. The approach affirms that the client at some level knows what she needs to focus on. The counsellor holds and communicates a facilitative attitude to create the therapeutic environment in which the client can have the opportunity to feel liberated to move more freely within herself and to experience and express what is present for her. The warm acceptance conveyed by the counsellor challenges any negative conditioning that might be associated with what the client then brings into the therapeutic relationship.

'Yes, and it is not just that, is it? I mean, there's what we have been exploring. The four-year-old me stubbornly digging her heels in and "busy me" trying to be like my mother.' Mandy shook her head. 'I just wish I could make sense of it all.'

Martin responded by handing back to what she had recognised for herself. 'So, your four-year-old being stubborn, your "busy me" copying your mother, your head saying go back to work, it makes you feel good, your heart questioning that but uncertain what it wants.' Martin was aware as he said the last few words that they were not a reflection of anything that Mandy had said, but he had noted that while her heart did seem to be saying 'change', she had not really indicated any sense of what this might be or mean. He added, 'You just wish you could make sense of it all.'

'Yes, and in a way it does make sense. Hearing you say back to me the gist of what I am saying, what I am thinking and feeling, really does make sense. It's where I am. It's like having conflicting demands made of me, but it is parts of me that are making the demands!'

'Parts of you, different parts of you, making conflicting demands.'

Mandy smiled, 'And I don't like having demands made of me, I don't like being told what to do. I can feel my four-year-old kicking off against it.' Mandy stopped and thought for a moment. 'You know, what I don't like is my head making demands of me. I think my head telling me to go back to work, telling me that it is good for me, is what this little girl in me is fighting against. She doesn't want to be told to go back to something that she can't cope with, or that makes her feel tired and. . . .' Mandy took in a deep breath and sighed loudly, blowing the air out of her mouth as she did so.

'Tired and. . . ?' Martin responded, wanting to help Mandy connect with and express with whatever had lay behind that deep sigh.

'Tired and fed up with it all. Fed up with the incessant demands, targets, deadlines, rushing around, keeping people happy, getting stuck in traffic, missing lunch breaks. I am fed up with it all. I want to find some peace. I want to do a job that I . . . I was going to say feel good about, but I know that part of me does feel good about my job. But another part of me doesn't, and I don't know what the answer is.' Mandy sighed again. She felt drained. She wanted to know what to do but she felt so torn by the conflicting voices inside her. She wanted them all to go away. Yet she knew as well that they were part of her and she needed to acknowledge this. She knew she had to get some clarity but at the moment she just felt terribly confused. She could hear Martin responding. He was saying, 'Fed up with so many things. You want some peace. You want to feel good about what you do.' She heard what he said, but in a way she wasn't really listening. She was wrapped up in her own thinking. Which part of me do I listen to? She didn't know. She was suddenly aware that it felt as if she had been a long time lost in thought.

'Sorry, I was miles away. Lost in thought. Now there's a way of summing it all up. But the more I think, the more confused I get. Yet I'm not sure that I can trust my feelings. I've always thought I was being logical. I thought that my work was a logical choice, and I know that work in a logical way. But look where it has got me. Yes, successful at marketing and managing my team, but at what cost to me?'

'At a cost to you,' Martin replied, offering a minimal empathic response so as not to disturb Mandy's flow.

'It has been at a cost to me. I have become too work-orientated, I have invested too much of me in my work. There's more to life. I need to make changes.'

'Need to make changes, yeah?' Again, Martin phrased his response as a question, offering the opportunity to Mandy to develop this further.

'And I want to say, yes, change my job, but I am aware that there is a hesitation in this. And I'm not sure what that is about.'

'A hesitation about change your job. Mhmm.'

'Mandy breathed deeply again, 'It doesn't feel right.'

Martin was unsure what didn't feel right. 'Doesn't feel right to change your job?'

'Yes and no. In many respects it makes so much sense to me to change my job, but I can also hear this little voice saying "so you change your job, but it'll still be you in the next job, still be the you with a stubborn four-year-old that doesn't want to be told what to do, still be a you that is struggling to claim her identity as a powerful woman, still be a you that is confused about who she is and what she wants''.'

Mandy is moving towards a recognition that changing is not going to be simply about what she does, but at least (and probably more) about changing her sense of self. People can rush into lifestyle changes on a surge of energy but without making the inner shifts that need to underpin them and which ensure that the changes are reflective of increasing congruence. However, changes that turn out not to be satisfying can be a valuable and important part of the process of resolving negative conditioning. As people redefine themselves and enter a process of recreating their sense, or structure, of self, they often need to experiment with change in order to truly discover what is most fulfilling for them. Mandy is recognising she must resolve her inner conflicts if she is to be sure that changes to work or other areas of her lifestyle are reflective of what *she* really wants. As yet, she it not clear in herself about herself.

'The little voice saying whatever job changes you make, you're still the same person underneath, still in conflict within yourself.' Martin could feel the struggle within Mandy. She looked somehow resigned to a struggle with herself. He was pleased, though, that she recognised this as she was clearly unlikely now to rush into changes that were without a firm foundation within herself.

'So I have to come to terms with me first of all, I have to. I have to learn to, well I suppose know myself well enough to be able to recognise why I make choices. I need greater self-awareness in all of this.' Mandy felt both excited and also anxious about all of this. As she spoke these words she both felt that it was within her reach and at the same time a huge step to take. 'Can I get to know myself well enough to really know what I want, what *I* really want, the whole me and not just a part of me that is like an echo from the past. I really want to free myself from feeling driven to be busy, to be successful, but I also recognise that I might still like to feel I can choose to be busy and seek success. It's this drive that I want to free myself from, the need that I thought was simply me but now I realise is a pattern from the past and that I have been subject to it.'

'What I am hearing, Mandy, is that you are recognising that you want to be free from this drive to be busy and successful, but that you may still want to strive for these things but not out of a need that, to use your words, "is an echo from the past".' Martin had noted Mandy had used the word 'successful', which he thought she hadn't mentioned before, and wondered if this urge was in some way slightly separate from the drive to be busy. It wasn't pressing, just a passing wonder, and he decided to keep it in the back of his mind, for now at least.

'Yes, I want to be free to make my own choices and to know that it is me, the whole me, the me that I am today, making that choice.'

'You want to be free so that the whole person that you are today is making choices,' Martin replied, maintaining and communicating his empathy for what Mandy had said.

'Yes, I want to be free.' Mandy stopped and smiled. 'I want to be free. Makes me think of that song Freddie Mercury sang. There's a line coming to mind, how does it go, something about being real?' She tried to remember, working her way through the song. 'Yes, that's it, "I've fallen in love for the first time and this time I know it's for real ...". I need to know myself for real. I think I'm getting there but I have further to go, don't I?'

'You want to know your self *for real.*' Martin spoke slowly and with deliberation, allowing the forcefulness and affirmative power of the words to be present and hopefully communicated to Mandy.

'I want to be the real Mandy, clear and open to who I am. I know I've been affected by my past, maybe I should say damaged by it all. I know it has left me with particular sensitivities, and maybe I don't yet know them all, but I want to feel able to be free to choose whatever I choose to do because I know it is what I, Mandy, the thirty-something-year-old woman, wants.'

That felt good, it felt energising and she also suddenly felt old. She felt as though time had gone by and she had been stuck somewhere. She shook her head slightly.

Martin sensed that Mandy was experiencing something different, her facial expression had changed. It had momentarily lost a kind of lightness that had been building up these last few minutes. 'You want to make choices as Mandy the thirty-something-year-old woman and I sense that something else has come to mind.'

'I suddenly felt old, as though life had rushed by and I was stuck somewhere in the past.' She shivered. 'I have to move on. I can't bury the past, I can't forget it. But I need to free myself from being uncontrollably subject to it.' She stopped and thought for a moment. Martin allowed her to continue her train of thoughts without interruption. 'I'm thinking about work. We haven't got round to looking at the pros and cons of staying or leaving, but I am realising that that does not matter. I have to know me and then I will know what to do. I can have all the advantages and disadvantages of staying or leaving in front of me, but it won't be which is the longest list that will drive my decision, it will be what I feel. That's what will be important, what I feel. At the moment I am not clear enough in myself to know what I feel, other than that I know I want some kind of change in my life.'

'What you *feel* is important to you, and you want clarity in yourself to know what you feel?' Martin responded, keeping to the recognition that was emerging for Mandy about her feelings.

'Yes, I need more time to really think about me, and I suppose to feel about me, though that sounds a bit odd. Phew, this is tiring stuff. I'm feeling energised and drained at the same time. I feel really enthralled by all of this, but I am aware that I am tired as well.'

Martin felt the urge to clarify what part of her was experiencing all of this. 'All of you is enthralled and all of you is tired, or part of you is enthralled and another part is tired?' he asked.

Mandy sat and thought about it. 'I'm not sure. There is an energy in all of this, and it feels good and my sense is that I need to stay with that and to kind of trust it somehow. But it is quite draining focusing on yourself. It takes a lot of concentration and I think I am beginning to lose that.'

Martin nodded and glanced at the clock. Just a few minutes before the end of the session. 'We only have a few minutes left. It feels like we have covered a lot today.'

'Yes, and it has helped consolidate for me the knowing that I am not yet securely in a place of complete self-awareness, but I am getting a clearer sense of who I am. But it is going to take time, and we only have two more sessions, yes?'

'Yes.'

'And there is no chance of any more?'

'No. six sessions is the maximum. It feels to me like we will have started a process, or rather, identified the process that had already started for you, affirmed and begun to clarify it. But the process will continue and you may need to work with it in other ways.'

'It feels a pity that I have to stop working with you.' Mandy could feel a sense of having to go through things again with someone else. She felt the rapport that she had with Martin, she trusted him and she didn't like the feeling of ending this with him.

Martin was aware of similar feelings. He also felt it a pity that counselling was limited. He knew what was coming next from Mandy because it did arise from time to time, and sure enough he heard her saying, 'Can I see you privately?'

'I'm afraid that in the NHS I can't do that. People have a right to treatment, and to continue seeing me outside of the NHS is like acknowledging that you have a need but the NHS is not offering you anything for it. Which is actually true, because that is what is happening. One option that we have is for you to take a break from counselling after six sessions and then ask the GP to refer you back to me at some point in the future.

'I'll think about that and see how I feel after we get to the end.'

'OK, we need to stop now, and we'll discuss options another time. Same time next week?'

'Yes, that will be fine. I'll see you then.' Mandy got up to leave, and Martin was left pondering his frustration at an NHS that rationed counselling and did not seem to appreciate that it could take people a lot of time to really change.

There are many ways of handling this situation. Where there is a rigid six-session rule, it can be argued that the matter should be referred back to the referring GP. A letter can be written by the counsellor and the client can then discuss his or her preferred course of action with the GP once the letter has been received. Continued work with the same counsellor has advantages, as a therapeutic relationship has been established and can provide the foundation for the ongoing work. The disadvantage is that it could be abused, with counsellors referring clients on to themselves for private work. By referring the matter back to the GP, a third party can be involved in the decision whether to refer the client on for private counselling, providing a safeguard against abuse.

Ideally, the number of sessions should not be rigid. There should be a build-in flexibility so that the service agreement is for an average number of sessions per client. Alternatively, and perhaps this is the most professional approach, the counsellors should simply be trusted as fellow professionals to make the decision in collaboration with clients as to how many sessions will be offered. This would, of course, be monitored as it could impact on waiting times, which might also be part of a service agreement. Often, it comes down to common sense and ensuring that the counsellor is employed working with client issues that are appropriate to their training and defined role.

Client case notes

Client acknowledged her need to make her own decisions as an adult woman in her own right, but is aware that childhood conditioning triggers her to push against being told what to do. She struggles to claim her identity as a woman with her own power, but by verbalising this realises greater strength. She has asked about further sessions with me outside of the NHS and I have said no and explained why.

Points for discussion/action

- Why do you think Mandy has not closed the shutter on Martin? What might he have done differently which could have provoked this in any of the sessions so far?
- Martin recognised he had directed Mandy after her comment concerning her four-year-old self sometimes being a strength and at other times getting in the way. Reflect on the value of being non-directive in therapeutic counselling.
- Must outer, practical changes always be underpinned by inner change and, if so, how does the person-centred approach encourage this?

- Does counselling ever enable us to forget or is it more the case that it enables clients to release themselves and redefine who they are in such a way that the hurt no longer stimulates incongruence?
- The counsellor draws attention to the client's body language at one point. How is this therapeutically helpful consistent with person-centred theory?
- Discuss the pros and cons of clients being offered private appointments to continue therapeutic work that has begun within the NHS.
- Critically evaluate Martin's work in this session from the standpoint of his application of the core conditions of empathy, congruence and unconditional positive regard.
- Make your own clinical notes of this session.

SUPERVISION 2

Martin had already spent some time with Anne briefly discussing two other clients before he turned to his work with Mandy. He was aware that his one-hour fortnightly supervision sessions were frequent enough to ensure that he had time to talk about his clients. He saw four clients a week at the surgery, most were weekly clients like Mandy, others fortnightly. He believed in being flexible and responsive to each client's needs. In fact, sometime he saw clients less frequently, particularly when they had problems making daytime appointments (he only worked during the day) due to work or other commitments. He had seen the odd client monthly, simply because their style was to want extra time between sessions to reflect on and apply insights they had gained through the counselling work.

It is important to be able to be flexible. People have different needs in relation to the difficulties that they bring to counselling. Some people may need a much more intense and supportive emphasis in the counselling they receive, others are looking for someone to talk through problems with and to formulate solutions.

The number of referrals and the level of counselling resources will govern, to a large extent, the length of waiting list that a counsellor may need to manage. Knowing that clients are waiting for appointments can be an added pressure. However, where a waiting list is due to a lack of resourcing of the service, this needs to be fed to those responsible for commissioning the service. Counsellors are employed to offer counselling and not to feel responsible for the limiting effect of under-resourcing.

The counsellor must also watch for under-resourcing affecting his work. The temptation can be to fit in extra clients for assessment only to find that consistent follow-up appointments are not possible. Clients who are engaged with should be offered an ongoing consistent service as agreed at the initial appointment.

Martin ensured that he at least mentioned each of his clients at each supervision session, even if he did not have a particular issue to explore.

'I want to move on to talk about Mandy now, Anne, as there have been some interesting developments and I feel I need to talk it through and get some feedback from you about the process. It has deepened again and I am still conscious of the limited number of sessions. This has come up, and I'll return to that later. What I want to focus on now is what she experienced in the session before last. I feel I need to talk it through as it was profound and powerful, and has helped Mandy understand more about what drives her. It has also generated problems for her as well, as she struggles to free herself from the effect of her early life.' Martin was looking thoughtful. There was something about Mandy that left him quite reflective, more so than with other clients.

'You look very thoughtful as you say all this, Martin, and I am curious. Your tone of voice has shifted from the way you were talking about your previous client. You seemed more animated somehow. Now, well, now it feels different. I don't know how it feels for you but I sense that there is a greater quietness and intensity.' Anne left her response at that and waited for Martin to pick up whatever felt most present and pressing.

'That's interesting.' Martin sat silently for a few moments. 'There is something that is leaving me thoughtful, although I am not aware of being this way in the sessions, or not particularly so. What I am touched by with Mandy is the powerful effect her childhood experience has had on her and my sense that we have hardly scraped the surface, yet we are already at the point of having to think about the ending of the counselling relationship.'

'So, the powerful effect of Mandy's childhood is what is causing you to be more thoughtful and reflective?' Anne responded, seeking to hold the focus on Mandy's impact on Martin as he had communicated it.

'Yes. Let me explain what happened in that third session. Quite unexpectedly, Mandy started talking about not wanting to do something, her voice changed and was very childlike and I really did not know what she was going to talk about. I could so easily have jumped into an assumption around sexual abuse when she said, ''please don't make me''. I didn't know what was coming next.' Martin paused for a moment and Anne responded.

'How did you respond to that, Martin?'

'I simply said in a quiet voice and with a hint of questioning, ''please don't make me?'' I was concerned not to say anything beyond what she had said, I wanted her to feel heard and to have a supportive and gentle space in which to continue if she wished. I wasn't sure whether she was speaking directly to me, but it didn't feel that way and the thought didn't cross my mind at the time. It felt as though her words were coming from very deep and from a long time ago. I was feeling very focused, as if all my senses had been tuned up. It felt like a huge moment, a significant moment in the therapy, and I just knew I had to be in that zone of heightened sensitivity and awareness.'

'You felt the importance and the significance.' Anne noted too how quiet it felt as she spoke. 'It feels quiet.'

Martin was feeling this too. He felt that somehow there was a need for reverence and respect for the client in the way that he and Anne talked about her. 'It was important and very significant. She had been talking about how busy she was and how this was linked back to her mother being busy. She then talked about not really knowing herself and feeling, how did she put it? Ah yes, as if she was "staring at some strange, new world", a world with "different rules or laws". She then added that she didn't know what these rules were or "how to be in that world". It was then that she said that she felt "very alone". I reflected back something like "you're facing a strange, new world, you're feeling very alone". Mandy went silent and tears appeared.'

Anne nodded and was aware that her own senses had heightened as well.

Martin continued. 'She began to look different, almost childlike. I asked her what she was feeling and it was then that she said "please don't make me". She then went on to talk as if she was aged four, about not wanting to be made to go to a Mr and Mrs Sharp who were going to foster her.'

Anne heard what Martin was saying about Mandy and she was also conscious of Martin and wanting to support him as he retold this part of the counselling session. 'How does this leave you feeling, Martin?' she asked.

Martin thought for a moment and reality-checked himself. What is present for me now, he thought? He voiced what was present for him as it came into his experience. 'I am feeling quiet. I have a sense of Mandy's powerlessness, of her smallness and it leaves me feeling small. But it also leaves me feeling very big and angry.'

Anne reflected back, seeking to use a tone of voice empathically reflecting what Martin had said. 'Quiet, powerless, small,' she deliberately spoke quietly as she said this. She then continued, 'yet also feeling very big and angry,' raising her tone of voice as she did so.

'Oh yes, very big and angry. But Mandy was small and powerless, she couldn't be a big, powerful and angry adult. I think she has struggled to be that ever since. She spoke with power in the session, but as I think about it now, I am aware that she hasn't shown much anger. In fact, I'm not sure that I can recall her being angry at all. I may be wrong on that, but thinking through as I sit here now nothing comes to mind.' Martin was trying to think back over the sessions, but nothing clear came to mind. Her claiming greater strength as a woman was present, that had been clear, but anger. She had talked about being angry at her foster parents but had not dwelt on that.

'So, Mandy is claiming power having felt very disempowered as a child, but no sense of anger being present?' Anne asked.

'I think it's present, it just hasn't come out. I think she must be sitting on a lot of anger and I think she showed this as a child, but my fantasy is that she learned not to be angry, either because it didn't change anything, or maybe things got worse and perhaps she was punished in some way. I don't know, these are my assumptions. She talked of hating her foster parents, of blaming them and blaming herself. I don't recall whether she used the word angry.

'So, your fantasy is that she is not showing anger for whatever reason, yes?'

'That's right. It's hard to be angry when you are powerless.' The words came out of Martin's mouth and he was struck by the forcefulness of this phrase. 'Wow, that came out with power, I wonder where that came from?'

Anne had noticed Martin's shift in tone. 'Sounds like it really came from you there?'

'Yeah, I really feel for Mandy, and hate the thought of her being shipped off like it seems that she was. That kind of gets to me. I guess I see a lot of clients who are struggling with the effects of their childhood and sometimes I guess it builds up.'

'Need to let some of it out now?' Anne asked. Then decided to add an empathic comment as a way of offering to hold Martin in his feelings. 'Children being treated like that really gets to you.'

'Yes, it does. It's so unnecessary and causes so many problems later in life. I always come back to asking why on earth do we not teach children parenting skills more in schools, I mean, it's the most important thing that we do as adults – well, I think it is – and how are we prepared for it? We learn from how we were treated, and we know the scale of abuse among children is horrendous.' Martin took a deep breath and could feel his eyes moistening. 'Just makes me bloody angry.' He knew he had raised his voice a little, he couldn't help it. He took in another deep breath. 'I needed to say that and to have it heard, Anne. It does build up and it is good to voice it and make it visible. I am affected by my work, I know I am, and it's because I care about the people I work with. I'm human. I'm touched by the stories I hear. And I'm glad to be able to come here and sound off about it. One of the really positive sides of counselling is the professional recognition of the need for supervision that encompasses the personal process of the professional.' Martin smiled, noting that his tension was easing. 'I can feel myself relaxing a little again so I want to move on.'

Working with people who have been affected at a very human level by experiences in their lives will impact on any professional who is working with them. This can be ignored and pushed away, many professions require this, but it has to go somewhere and can often sit within the professional and affect his reactions to clients. Having a place and space to let some of this go, where it builds up, ensures safer practice and the health and wellbeing of the professional concerned. It ensures that the counsellor can remain feeling human otherwise he would need to start protecting himself from his own feeling reactions, which would make it difficult for him to be fully and authentically present for his clients, a crucial factor in counselling, particularly where there is a strong relational component as is the case with the PCA.

Anne knew that Martin was affected by his work and she agreed with him that this was a strength and not a weakness. Good counselling, in her opinion, included the very human factor of two people meeting person to person. Where this occurred, both were affected. She recognised, too, that in a therapeutic approach that recognised and utilised the power of relationship, this was perhaps an even more significant factor.

'So, what do you want to move on to? Anything further with Mandy?'

'Yes, there was something that came up in the last session where she was struggling to claim her power as a woman. I got caught on trying to respond empathically to something she said.'

'Tell me more,' Anne replied, with genuine interest and curiosity.

'Mandy was struggling to claim her power as a woman and at one point said, "I am a woman", and, well as a man it felt weird saying, "I am a woman", a straight reflection. But I also didn't feel at ease with saying "you are a woman" either. I remember thinking that had I been a woman myself I may not have had this dilemma.'

'So, your sense is that had you been a woman you could have made the straight reflection and felt comfortable with it?'

'Yes, it would have somehow felt right, but it didn't. My sense of my own gender identity got in the way. But to say "you are a woman" didn't feel right.'

'So, where were you when this was happening?' Anne asked, aware of a sense that Martin had lost the client somewhere.

'Where was I? What do you mean?' Martin wasn't sure what Anne was getting at.

'Well, where was your focus? Who were you focusing on in all of this?'

'Well, Mandy. I was trying to find the words to reflect empathically what she had said.'

'So in those moments you were thinking about the right words to say?'

'Ye-es,' Martin replied, feeling a little hesitant and wondering where Anne was heading.

'Where were you looking for those words, Martin?'

Martin thought for a moment. A smile broke out across his face. 'In me. I wasn't in the client's frame of reference, was I? I got tangled up in myself and my own reaction. That's really interesting and helpful, because what I wanted to come on to, was a little bit later I actually did reflect back the words "you are a woman" and they came out sounding right and natural, utterly spontaneously.'

'So you spent time thinking about it and being undecided what to say and how to say it, and in the end said nothing. But when you let go of that dilemma the words just flowed out and felt right. Is that how it was?' Anne asked.

'Yes, and it really was quite a contrast. I'm sure if I had said something when I was struggling it just wouldn't have had the same therapeutic value as when I did reflect back "you are a woman".' Martin was shaking his head. 'It is amazing. Same words but my sense is that had they not been spoken from some sort of spontaneous focus it just would not have worked. I can't be sure, of course, but that is my sense.'

'It seems to me that the spontaneity was somehow key in all of this, and that this was itself an expression of the connection that was established between you and Mandy.'

'I just didn't think, I was in kind of free fall.'

Martin found himself wondering about what part congruence and incongruence had played in this interaction with Mandy. When he had hesitated, had he been in an incongruent state and therefore not accurately in touch with himself, or for that matter with Mandy? But when the words had spontaneously emerged, perhaps there had been a shift that had enabled him to regain his own congruent focus and a deeper sense of connection with Mandy.

It struck him how one might say the same thing to a client, but the power of what is said is more connected with where it comes from rather than the actual words themselves. This was not easy to describe, and might not be understood by someone observing an interaction. In a sense, only the counsellor and the client could fully appreciate and experience the relational dynamics that underlay a particular empathic response and the role of congruence in ensuring that the words spoken were free and authentic.

'You look thoughtful, Martin,' Anne commented, noting that he had been quiet and frowning a little.

'Yes, I was pondering the significance of being empathic and congruent. In many ways I can think of these as being somehow in competition. Can I be empathic to my client if I am attending to my own authenticity, and conversely, can I be authentically and expressive of me when my focus is within the client's frame of reference? I think we kind of dance between the two, and yet I am wondering now if there is not a depth of communication which kind of includes yet transcends both empathy and congruence.'

Anne was intrigued. 'Go on.'

'Well, can we actually be both and if so, what happens in that moment? It must surely be that deep connection when there is a true meeting of persons, a moment that I would describe as simply one of deep knowing. But I don't want to get into that now as I have other clients I want to talk about today. I feel I have gained a lot from what we have been exploring, but I am aware of the time and I have other themes I want to address.'

'You get me intrigued by something and then you move on, like holding out a cake and just as I have decided to take a bite out of it and experience it, you pull it away! But, yes, I am mindful of the time. Maybe this idea of transcending yet somehow including congruence and empathy in the moment is one to explore another time. It fascinates me but I am aware that you have other topics and clients to focus on. So let's move on.'

Points for discussion/action

- Has Martin addressed all the issues that need addressing from the previous two sessions and, if not, what might he also have explored?

- Much of the supervision session has addressed Martin's feelings. What is the value of this in supervision?
- How would you feel had you been Martin at the end of the supervision session?
- Critically evaluate the supervision session from the angle of person-centred working?

Mandy had phoned in to the surgery two days earlier. She had been taken ill. She
did not expect to be able to make it to the session that week and wanted to
ensure that the surgery were aware in case they could reallocate her time that
week to someone else. The surgery had passed this on to Martin.

How do counsellors react to clients cancelling or not attending appointments? For trainees this can be quite a difficult experience. As in this case,
clients will phone to cancel. Sometimes the reason given will feel perfectly
valid and reasonable to the counsellor. At other times they might feel
aggrieved that something else has been chosen in spite of the counselling
agreement to meet. Obviously, where the latter is the case the counsellor
may wish to address this, particularly if it remains a persistent thought in
his mind as he seeks to work with the client in the next session.

From the person-centred perspective, the client will have the freedom
to choose her focus for the next session, and the counsellor will raise
the matter of the cancelled or non-attended appointment in response to the
need for authenticity and transparency within the relationship.

Where a client does not attend for a first appointment, the response may
be governed by the service protocol. Perhaps a second appointment will be
offered or a letter will be sent asking the client to contact the surgery to confirm her wish for a further appointment. Alternatively, the GP could be
informed and a joint decision taken as to which response to make.

Where a client does not attend with no word, after having attended a session or sessions, it can impact on the counsellor, leaving him with feelings
such as abandonment, anger or self-doubt. This can be particularly so for
the trainee or newly qualified counsellor. These feelings will need acknowledging in supervision to ensure that where strong feelings are triggered that
have hooked into issues that are the counsellor's, this strength of feeling is
not carried back into the counselling session.

Martin asked the receptionist to call Mandy back and confirm her time for the following week. He also agreed that if the GPs had anyone else they wanted

assessed for counselling, they could refer them in to that time slot. His decision to agree to this was based on the fact that he knew Mandy's six sessions would end soon and that this would open up a regular slot for someone else. He tried to avoid giving people initial sessions knowing that they would then have a potentially long wait before he could see them again and preferred to offer a more consistent and regular series of sessions.

Managing referrals and allotting appointment times is handled in many different ways. There is no right or wrong way. Many counsellors have evolved systems that best suit the culture of the surgery. Sometimes, the receptionist books people into available slots, sometimes the GPs. In other instances, referral letters are sent to the counsellor who makes contact with the clients and books them in. All of these ensure scope for a degree of fast response for clients to be offered appointments.

However, with more counselling services becoming part of primary care trusts or mental health trusts, centralisation can have the effect of slowing down the process so that response times are longer, with referrals being sent into a central pool, then allocated to particular counsellors who then contact the clients.

In fact, a locum GP did refer someone in for an initial assessment/counselling session, and the client was seen. However, this turned out to be an inappropriate referral. The client was very vulnerable and suicidal and Martin, and the client, felt that he needed more intense ongoing support from a community mental health team (CMHT). This was communicated to the GP, who made the referral to the CMHT. The GP had not appreciated that there was a protocol as to what issues the counsellor was allowed to work with under the service agreement.

Therapeutic counsellors are trained to work with a variety of issues, and may feel able to work with material that is outside their role within a surgery. Where this arises, it will need to be discussed either with the referring GP or the trust or agency that provides the counselling service. The areas that some counselling service agreements may prohibit counsellors from working with can include drugs and alcohol, sexual abuse issues, clinical depression, suicidal ideation, personality disorder and eating disorders.

Generally material that is not contained within a counselling service agreement is that which specialist services may be available to respond to (addiction, eating disorder, mental health) or issues that will clearly require more than a time-limited response can offer.

Martin had spent a lot of time at the surgery helping GPs and other members of the primary healthcare team to understand what counselling actually was. It is a fact of life that most professionals who have done a counselling skills training will say they offer counselling to clients. Yet this is unlikely to be the kind of therapeutic counselling that a qualified counsellor will be offering. The trained counsellor will have had to undergo rigorous training in a particular model, or models, and achieve a degree of personal growth either through the training process and/or through personal therapy, which will have prepared him for deeper work with clients.

As a person-centred counsellor, Martin had sought to stress to other members of the surgery team the relational quality of the counselling work that he offered, and how it differed from the more prescriptive culture of medicine. He had managed to convey the fact that the way he worked did not have a specific goal that he set prior to the sessions, but rather that his goal was to create a therapeutic climate in which the attitudinal qualities of congruence, empathy and unconditional positive regard could be present, communicated and hopefully received by the client. At first, the GPs had been a little sceptical, seeing counselling as a treatment to be prescribed to patients. But they had come round as they saw the value of this approach in helping people to re-evaluate their lives and experiences, and redefine themselves as a result of feeling listened to and valued by the counsellor.

Martin had introduced a system of feedback forms for clients to complete, which he drew from in his annual report. These were a combination of quantitative and qualitative questions. By far the most common response was that the clients, while initially apprehensive, felt relieved that they had someone to talk to, and that what was of value was to have time in which to make sense of themselves and to make choices about their lives without having someone with a heavy agenda.

Mandy would have been Martin's final client that day. As he prepared to leave the surgery he was aware that he was thinking about her and hoping that the heavy cold which had stopped her attending would soon clear up. He had been looking forward to working with her. He found the content of the sessions challenging but very moving. Only two more sessions with her, he thought, not a lot of time to address the issues that she has from early life and to help her make decisions in the present and for the future that would be right for her.

The GP who had referred Mandy happened to be passing the counselling room and popped her head round the door. 'How's Mandy doing?'

GPs have a duty of care towards their patients and will often expect to be kept informed. However, counsellors are working to a confidentiality contract with clients that generally will limit what can be disclosed to other parties, including their GP. Some counsellors will be quite clear in keeping a rigid boundary, others will convey general information without disclosing content when asked in this way.

Martin smiled. He was not going to refuse to say anything as he knew that was unhelpful, and he knew that the GP was genuinely concerned for Mandy's wellbeing. She was a GP who often referred clients and did appreciate the boundary issues around confidentiality.

'She's doing well. It hasn't been easy for her, and she has a lot of material to work with from those early experiences that you mentioned to me. I think six sessions may be too short, but we will be discussing this and exploring options. I don't feel I can say much more due to confidentiality on the content of the sessions.'

'I appreciate that. I don't want to put you in an awkward position.' Dr Hill smiled. 'She had been so upset when I saw her that time before referring her to you. She's still off work. I don't want her rushing back before she is ready.'

'No, that would be a mistake. I'm sure she will want to discuss that with you when her current sick certificate runs out.' Martin didn't feel he was saying anything out of place.

'Fine. I'll discuss it with her then. It is a problem having only six sessions with people. I think we have learned from this and next year we are going to be more flexible.'

Martin recognised the temptation to say more about how Mandy might benefit from more sessions, but recognised that he had not had permission from her to discuss this with Dr Hill, that she had wanted to think about her options and discuss them during their final session. So he kept his comments general.

'Yes, I agree. I think it has to be either on an average number of contacts or we discuss it with you whenever a client and myself feel a need for further sessions.'

'OK. Well, I'm glad counselling is helping Mandy. Must dash, about to start surgery. See you next week.'

'Yes, bye.' Martin picked up his file of notes and returned them to the filing cabinet, which he locked. He recognised that he felt good working in primary healthcare. He had seen it change as counselling became more understood and accepted. He had seen how the GPs had come, not exactly to rely on it, but they were certainly aware of not wanting to lose it. So many patients needed the time they could not give, and the expertise in enabling them to address the problems that had arisen for them. He was always amazed at the range of issues, although low mood, anxiety and stress were by far the most common symptoms his clients presented with. Of course, the underlying causes were wide-ranging and often the GP was unaware of these, the patient having not disclosed them, or simply not made the connection to them.

He paused for a moment and reflected on the issues that recent clients had been referred to him with: marital problems, work-related stress, low self-esteem, panic attacks, loss of job, being thrown out of home, abusive neighbours, a wife struggling to cope with her recently retired husband, bereavement, fears of various kinds. One thing was sure, there was very little predictability in this job. He liked the variety. But most of all, he owned the fact that he enjoyed working with people and the feeling that he could help them make a positive difference in their lives. It was a good feeling. But he also recognised that however much of a vocation counselling can be, it is still a job, and he was careful to ensure that he had other interests in his life. He believed in balance and in ensuring that, as far as possible, he could gain a sense of satisfaction through a variety of experiences. What was it tonight? Oh yes, salsa. Get him into his body and out of his head for a couple of hours at least, and give his feelings a bit of an exhilarating boost as well!

> Martin has wisely recognised that he needs balance in his life to ensure his own emotional and mental wellbeing. Each counsellor will make his own choices. However, time for recreation is important. The constant exposure to emotional problems is debilitating. Supervision will help to some degree, as may personal therapy, but other non-therapeutic interests and involvement can be a necessity.

Client case notes

Client cancelled her appointment as she was unwell. She plans to attend next week. Conversation with Dr Hill. Told her the client was doing well but had a lot of material from early childhood to deal with.

Points for discussion/action

- Design a protocol giving details of what issues clients should be referred to a community mental health team for, and which issues would appropriately be handled by a surgery counsellor.
- Was Martin right to make any disclosure about Mandy to the GP?
- How might you react to a GP requesting information informally about a client?
- Design a feedback questionnaire for clients to complete at the end of a series of counselling sessions.
- Formulate your own notes for Mandy's non-attendance.

SESSION 6

Martin's previous client had been very distressed at the end of her session and he was pleased that he gave himself 15 minutes between appointments. It had been quite an emotional session and he had felt very drained at the end. He had jotted down his notes, which he would write up later. He kept his own notes in his client file at the surgery and he put a very brief comment on one of the patient cards in the surgery notes. This was never detailed but simply provided the GP with information as to whether the client was attending and what was discussed in general terms. So he might write: 'family issues explored', 'focus on work-related difficulties', 'explored plans for the future', 'mood lifting a little'.

He decided to go for a quick walk. It was cool outside and he felt he needed some fresh air and a few minutes to collect his thoughts and let go of some of the feelings that he had been left with. He generally found that a quick walk around the block – it took no more than five minutes – helped him to regain his focus.

Time between clients is vital and good practice. Counsellors should resist moves to 'conveyor belt' clients. Too much of the medical profession is based on moving people through back to back. It is unhealthy for professionals and for clients or patients, who often feel rushed and may therefore find it difficult to say what they want to say. Others might accuse counsellors of being precious, but counsellors should be trained to know how to look after themselves and to ensure their own psychological health and well-being as part of their professional practice.

Counsellors need time to clear themselves sufficiently of their reactions, feelings and thoughts in order to be appropriately present for their next client. A person-centred counsellor, for whom congruence and empathy are crucial features of effective counselling, will need to have given themselves preparation time. Issues held over from a previous client can obstruct both congruence and empathy, and distract the counsellor from giving the next client the focused attention that she has a right to expect.

As he walked Martin deliberately chose to focus on what he was experiencing in his body. He liked to feel the cool air that he was breathing in and the feel of movement as he walked along. He liked to look around and just allow his senses to be open to the stimulation around him. He often felt that the counselling room dampened down some of his more physical senses and he wanted to breath vitality back into himself.

On his return he took a glass of cool water, and brought one in to the counselling room for Mandy in case she wanted it. He then spent a moment sitting with his eyes closed, just composing himself and allowing himself to simply be present. He opened his eyes and looked at the clock just as he heard a tap on the door and the receptionist telling him that his last client had arrived.

Mandy walked into the room and Martin immediately noticed that she seemed somehow a little more self-assured. He hadn't really thought that she wasn't confident, but there was something different about her today. He decided to convey his experience to her.

'You look to me as though you are a little more self-assured.'

'Yes, I do feel more confident somehow. I'm still off work but I have talked it through with the GP and I have persuaded her to let me go back next week. I want to see how I get on before ending the counselling, so I can talk about what happens when I see you next time.' Mandy had decided that while she had some mixed feelings about going back, she wanted to see how she reacted and still have time to talk it through with Martin. She had come to counselling today with the intention of talking through what might happen, how she might handle it, and what her options were.

Martin knew he wasn't sure about Mandy going back too quickly, but he also respected her right to make her own choices. He was ready to support her in her decision, though he was a little uneasy given the powerful impact that her past experiences had had upon her. Nevertheless, she had made a decision and no doubt this was satisfying a part of her nature. He didn't want to undermine her by questioning her decision, but he was prepared to help her explore it more fully so she had a clear sense of what was happening for her.

'So, back next week.' He tried to say it without sounding concerned, or being too upbeat either. He realised the fact that he was trying to say it in a particular way smacked of incongruence. The fact was that he was uneasy and maybe he did need to voice this. But he didn't want to implant doubt in Mandy's mind about her decision. He decided to hold back on expressing his feelings and thoughts, and rather maintain his empathic focus on Mandy.

Martin is being incongruent but he is not clear why. He is experiencing unease but is unable to voice this. He effectively gives himself a reason for not voicing it by deciding to focus on his empathy for Mandy. This is later explored in supervision, which brings to light what might be happening for Martin, blocking him from being authentic.

Whenever a counsellor experiences an unease about something they have said, or not said, it is worth taking this to supervision. The reasons behind the unease may not be obvious, but can have far-reaching effects on client work. It is important for counsellors to know themselves sufficiently clearly in order to be able to pick up on moments or even periods within the counselling session where they sense they may be lacking

'Yes. Well, I gave it a lot of thought, and being laid up with that cold also gave me more time to just think about things. I have realised a great deal about myself in these sessions, and I know that the past has affected me. I hope that I will be returning a little wiser. I also feel as though I don't want to rush into anything, but I do feel more open to alternative possibilities. I guess I want to keep my options open.'

'Mhmm,' Martin added after a pause, 'so, you have gained a great deal of self-awareness and you don't want to rush into anything. You want to keep your options open.'

'I do. I mean, it may be too soon, I'm really not sure about that, but I kind of feel I want to see what happens. And I want to be able to talk it through at the next session.' Mandy knew that she wasn't totally convinced, but she felt that she had a better understanding of herself and what was driving her to work and succeed, and to be busy. But she felt she could now step away from this a little. Of course, whether she could under the pressure and stress of work was another matter, but she felt she wanted to give it a go.

'So part of you feels it may be too soon but you want to see what happens and have the opportunity to discuss it here next week.'

'Yes, I have spoken to my manager, who is happy with me having the afternoon off for the counselling session next week. I think he was glad I was coming back. He said that they had missed me. But I'm not sure that they will be getting the same person back, somehow.'

'Not the same person?' Martin reflected the words back to Mandy with a questioning tone, curious as to what difference she was anticipating and wanting her to have the opportunity to affirm it.

'I know that the way I was, simply does not work for me. I thought it did. Being busy, rushing around, taking things on, yes, it did make me feel good. But it didn't work in the long run. I wasn't managing myself. I was just reacting, saying yes to everything. I wasn't thinking, or if I did, that need to be busy, to somehow justify myself, kept driving me on.'

The words *justify myself* stood out for Martin, and he reflected them back, again with a hint of questioning in his voice. 'Justify yourself?'

Sometimes, as in this case, words used by a client can stand out sharply. The counsellor may not have any distinct knowledge of why this may be so. Again, the counsellor needs the level of self-awareness that will enable him to discern whether the words have particular meaning for him and therefore may have less significance for the client, or whether they do not convey particular meaning within the counsellor's frame of reference and are therefore more likely to have significance for the client. In cases where the words stand out and have significance for the counsellor, the response will be to own this, for instance 'Hearing you say ... has meaning for me but I am wondering whether it has special meaning for you.' Where the counsellor does not sense any significance within his frame of reference, he is more likely, as in the above text, to simply reflect them back to the client and allow the client space to respond.

'Needing to be busy, needing to prove something.'
Martin continued with his questioning tone, gently holding Mandy and allowing her to continue to elaborate on her theme. 'Prove something?'
'Yes, I needed to prove....,' Mandy hesitated for a moment, not liking the words that had come to mind.
Martin had noticed an anxious look spread fleetingly across her face. He simply moved his head slightly and raised his eyebrows a little as if to say, 'Yes, tell me more.'

Empathy is not only communication by words. Body language can be extremely effective in encouraging a client to say a little more about something, particularly as in this case where the communication from the client has been through the body. However, as with all forms of communication, there is the risk of a misinterpretation and the counsellor should bear this in mind.

Mandy smiled, but it felt an uncomfortable smile. He doesn't miss anything, she thought. She took a deep breath. 'I needed to prove that I was good enough.'
'Needed to prove you were good enough. That seemed really difficult to say.'
'I guess it's that sense of not being good enough that made me uncomfortable. It isn't something I normally dwell on. I suppose I'm always too busy to really think about this kind of thing. But yes, I do feel I need to prove myself to be good enough.'
Martin was wondering who she needed to prove this to. It was quite a strong wonder and he decided to voice it. 'I am wondering who you needed to prove yourself to.'
'Myself,' was Mandy's rapid answer to that question, but in truth she had also felt another word come strongly to mind, 'mother'. But she did not voice it.

Mandy is thinking one thing but saying something else. She is being incongruent, probably in order to avoid immediate discomfort, or disclosing something that she senses might lead her to discomfort. In a sense it is a form of denial, however denial is often misrepresented in a negative manner. In fact, the client is simply being how she needs to be in that moment, seeking to preserve some semblance of wellbeing and avoid hurt. We all do this. Denial is not pathological but a normal human reaction to feeling ashamed, guilty, uncomfortable. It indicates that the client has feelings about something, strong feelings that drive her into incongruence and a heightened state of anxiety that, paradoxically, actually generates further discomfort. People will deny something until they perceive that the risk of disclosure is less uncomfortable than the struggle to preserve the fiction.

'So, you have been proving to yourself that you are good enough. Good enough for what?'

'I don't know, I suppose it is the childhood stuff again. I didn't really adjust well to being with my foster parents. When I started school I didn't want to be there and so I didn't really try to mix with other children. It was quite a lonely time. I didn't do too well. I remember being told I was a disruptive little girl and that I should know better. I can still see the teacher as she said that to me. But I didn't care. At least, I thought I didn't care, but thinking about it now I am sure that I did. I don't know what I wanted then, maybe I was attention seeking, may be I was just. . . , oh, I don't know. I was just another lonely kid who hadn't got her own way and I suppose in my own way wanted everyone to know about it.'

'So it was a lonely time, you can remember the teacher and being told you were disruptive and should know better, you're not sure whether or not you really cared, but you have a sense of wanting everyone to know that you hadn't got your way.' Martin had decided to offer back a fuller reflection. There had been so many different elements in what Mandy had said and he didn't want to direct her to any one part of it all.

Mandy sat quietly for a moment, reflecting on the words that Martin was repeating back to her. It all seemed so long ago, she had few distinct memories, but she did remember the teacher's face, and the tone of her voice. She had hated it. She was aware she had taken a deep breath as she thought that. She hadn't connected with that before.

'I hated how that teacher spoke to me. But I couldn't help being how I was. I got bored very easily. I never could sit down for very long! Even then I. . . ,' Mandy paused again. She shook her head. 'Even then I was busy all the time.'

'Mhmm. Busy all the time and hated the way the teacher had spoken to you.'

'I was busy, but that was way before I was back with my mother and seeing her being busy all the time. I mean, what we had been talking about before had left me thinking I had picked this busy-ness thing up from her. Well maybe in some ways I did, in association with work. But now I think about it I was on the go all the time long before that.' Mandy paused and thought again. 'What's that condition kids have these days, you know, where they can't keep attention on anything for long, attention deficit disorder, isn't it? Well, maybe I had that. I don't know. But I was certainly a restless child.' Mandy could feel herself experiencing an unease at this insight. While thinking her drive to do had been a trait she had copied from her mother had been difficult to accept, it had at least left her feeling she could change it and learn to be different, to be how she wanted to be. But if her busy-ness was somehow genetic, nature rather than nurture, what then?

Martin's empathy has enabled Mandy to explore and expand on her theme. The longer empathic response which summarised what Mandy had said was then followed up later with a much shorter empathic response, helping Mandy to focus in on what was important for her. This then leads her to expand more fully on the tendency to be busy and to engage with a dilemma over whether her busy-ness can be changed. This in turn leads her to engage with her strong feelings and determination to search for, know and be herself.

Martin was aware from the frown on her face that Mandy was thinking. She hadn't said anything though.

'You're frowning.'

'Mhmm? Oh yes. I just had a rather uncomfortable thought. I mean, if my need to be busy came from being conditioned into it by seeing how my mother was, well, I could change that. I would need to step back from that and discover how I need to be, you know, the me that is me. Oh that sounds crazy, but I know what I mean.'

Martin decided to respond and try to let Mandy know what he was hearing her say. 'Yeah, to step back from the conditioned you and rather be the you that is free of all that, the kind of unconditioned you?'

'Yeah, me. God, so much of these sessions seem to keep coming back to me, to some kind of search to discover who I am and to be that person.' She breathed in deeply and sighed as she let out the breath. She felt a little tired by it all, and at the same time she knew that she had to stay with it.

'A search to be you,' Martin responded, sharpening up the emphasis a little.

'A search to be me. But who am I? Last time I was really struggling to own myself as a woman. What kind of woman? I realise I am a woman with power, my own power, but power to do what? I don't want to use it to get locked back into a cycle of busy-ness all over again. And what had begun to freak me out just now was the thought that my drive to be busy might be genetic, be who I really am, and that I am powerless to change it. Can you change your genes?' Mandy's eyes had widened a little as she had said this, and she really was feeling a sense of helplessness.

'The way you say it makes it sound scary.' Martin wasn't too sure whether he was saying this as an empathic response to how he sensed Mandy was feeling, or whether it was his own stuff. He wasn't sure whether it had been a helpful thing to say, but he had said it now.

'It is scary. I don't want to feel that I cannot change. I really don't.'

Martin noticed that Mandy's eyes had moistened a little. 'You really don't feel that you want to change. Really strong feelings.'

Mandy could feel herself going quiet as she nodded. Oh God, she thought, I was determined not to be tearful again this session, but focus on my work and how to handle it. She reached over for a tissue and dabbed at her cheeks and ran the edge of the tissue around her eyelids, trying to avoid smudging her mascara.

'I want to change. I want to feel more in control. I want to feel . . . to feel as though I have my hands on the controls, you know? I don't want to feel driven by my mother's style of working, or by some genetic urge that I have no control over. I just want to be. . . ,' Mandy hesitated again.

Martin reflected back to try and help Mandy verbalise what she was experiencing, and using the first person to make it more powerful for Mandy to hear. 'I just want to be. . . .'

'I just want to be normal. I just want to feel I am being who I really am. And I want to be comfortable with myself as well. I was never really that comfortable as a child, well, I suppose I've only felt comfortable in my work, in being busy.'

Martin reflected back the last few words, although he was profoundly aware of how little he knew about Mandy in terms of what she did to relax, or even if she ever did relax. He noted the wonder and put it to one side, deciding to voice it only if it persisted. 'Only felt comfortable being busy.'

Martin could have let his curiosity get the better of him, but he has kept his focus and pushed aside any fleeting need to know that he may have had. If Mandy wants him to know about how she relaxes, she will tell him. His role as a person-centred counsellor is to be attentive to what she wishes to communicate to him. He will only ask questions where the question is persistent and is sensed to have relevance to what is present within the therapeutic relationship. Simply wanting information out of curiosity is not justification when working to a person-centred model.

'Yes. I'm not good at relaxing. I tend to be busy even then, doing things in the garden, being on a couple of committees in the village. I suppose I don't really relax. But I have been the last few weeks, I've had to. I just haven't had the energy to do much. I haven't wanted to do much, and that isn't me. And yet somehow, I have accepted it. That seems strange, somehow. I mean, surely I should have found it really uncomfortable not being able to do anything?'

'You look really surprised at that,' Martin replied.

'I would have expected to have found it difficult. But it hasn't been. But I really haven't had the energy. Maybe not having the energy has made it more easy. But my energy level has begun to pick up a little the last few days, since I had that heavy cold last week. And it was then that I decided to go back to work.' Mandy took a deep breath. 'Dammit, here I go again. A little bit of energy and here I am planning to go back to work, back to being busy, busy, busy.'

Mandy looked very fired up, and full of emotions. He decided to empathise and spoke with a little extra fire in his voice. 'Fires you up with a lot of feeling, yeah?'

'Sure does. I mean, what is it about me?' Mandy had raised her voice and was shaking her head. 'But I know that I am not going to go back as the person I was. I am determined to be different. I want to be in control. I don't want to make the same mistake of overdoing it. Yet it feels so difficult to get rid of something that feels so much a part of me.' Mandy was looking, and sounding, quite angry.

'You sound quite angry with yourself, Mandy.' Martin spoke the words quite briskly, seeking to maintain the momentum that Mandy had established as she had been speaking.

An example of empathy reflecting not just the words but the tone and the feelings associated with what is being communicated. This allows the client to escalate her tone a little more, perhaps helping her to engage with and communicate more fully and accurately what she is experiencing. It is helping the client to become more authentic, and to experience the power and satisfaction that comes from this.

'I am angry, and frustrated. I really want to get a grip on myself. I really want to slow down, to relax. I really do, and I'm bloody well determined to achieve it. I know I have to change. I've got to watch out for constantly sliding back into that old pattern. It's like a rut that you get into but you don't realise you are in it. You rush up and down it but all the time it gets deeper and deeper, until you forget that there is anything beyond your little rut. Well, it's time to climb out of it and keep away from it.'

'You sound pretty clear and determined to me. You're going to get out and stay out of that damn rut.' Martin had again used a strong tone of voice.

'Yes, I am.' Mandy paused again. She had suddenly been struck by a sense of not being too sure what life would be like outside of her rut. It suddenly struck her the immensity of the change she was contemplating. 'It's not just about work, is it? I've got to change other things as well.' She spoke quite quietly. She brought her hands up to her mouth and blew out a deep breath. 'OK, I've got to start thinking this through. Genetic or not, I have to make changes to this drive to be busy, to justify myself, to be good enough, whatever. That's got to go. I have to move on. I have to make choices for me and try to ensure that these choices don't send me back into that rut.'

Martin was aware of nodding as he listened to Mandy. She was doing a good job in affirming her needs without his need to say very much. She was in full flow, or so it felt to him.

Mandy was continuing. 'OK, so I need some strategies here. I need to look at my work and my leisure time and figure out how I am going to give myself a chance to be different.' Mandy suddenly felt a wave of self-consciousness sweep over her. 'Sorry, I seem to be talking a lot.'

'Seems to me you are saying a lot of important things, things that maybe you need yourself to hear.'

'Yes, but I do want to think about some practical stuff. Particularly about work. But I'm not sure where to start.'

'OK, so practical stuff, how to keep out of that busy rut when you are at work, yes?'

'Yes.'

Martin has honoured Mandy's wish to focus on some practical strategies. He had initially responded to Mandy by communicating his sense that she was saying important things that maybe she needed to hear, and this might have held her with this focus if she had wanted this. But this was not the case. She feels in need of strategies and repeats this. Martin acknowledges this but is careful to give the lead back to Mandy.

'So, what comes to mind?'

Mandy thought for a moment. What really gets to me about work? 'Not being able to say "no" to demands that take over my day and my evenings sometimes.'

'You want to hear yourself saying "no" a little more often, yes?'

'I do, and I want it to be an appropriate "no". We talked before about how stubborn I can be when I am pushed. I can feel that if I'm not careful I might start saying "no" to everything. I don't want that either. I need some kind of balance. Well, maybe not balance, it is more a case of appropriateness. I want to feel able to say no when it is appropriate to say no, when demands are being made of me that I genuinely feel are unrealistic.'

'Can you give examples?' Martin realised he wasn't being directly empathic but he felt that some concrete examples might help to anchor more clearly what Mandy wanted to change, and he was mindful that she had said earlier that she wanted some practical ideas.

'My manager is always good at wanting updated figures on sales at short notice. Often he'll say the day before some meeting that he needs them next morning. He's known to not plan ahead, and I suppose in a way we collude with that because, well, I can't speak for others, but I end up running around like a headless chicken, getting figures from my team and frantically putting them together and into a report. It's crazy. He must know he needs these figures.'

'OK, so he leaves it to the last minute and you end up like a headless chicken.'

'Yes, and it is ridiculous. Why can't he get his bloody act together and get off my case. Bastard.' Mandy spoke these words with tremendous force and emphasis. She suddenly grinned. 'That felt good!'

Martin smiled back. 'Anything else?'

'All he ever seems to think about are targets. I know they're important, but we do have a big turnover in staff. Many people don't stay. In fact, I've been there as long as anyone really. I seem to be constantly travelling around to my team, as well as chasing my own customers and meeting new and potential clients as well. The miles I do.'

'So you go round to each of your team, yes? How often?' Martin could feel a sense of wonder as to whether Mandy had to do *all* the running around, but he didn't want to suggest it. He rather hoped she would start to question her own style of management.

'I have to see each of them each week, and there are eight in the team. We discuss what is coming up for them each week.'

'So you go round to each of them.' Martin deliberately spoke slowly.

'Yes. It takes up at least two days of my week, sometimes more. It's ridiculous.'

'Mhmm. It's ridiculous.' Martin let the silence hang as Mandy thought about it.

'Why do I have to do all the running around? My manager has a team of managers like me, he doesn't run around like I do.'

'He doesn't. . . ,' Martin didn't have time to finish.

Mandy continued, 'So why should I?' She paused and thought. 'They could come to me. Maybe not every week, but they could come to me more than they do. At the moment we all get together every six weeks, maybe I should change this to every three or four weeks. That would be a start. And it might be good for a bit more team-building as well. It might help them feel a little more part of the organisation. It can feel quite lonely sometimes when you spend a lot of time "on the road".' Mandy thought about it. 'Yes, I'll suggest that and get it up and running. OK, so that's one change I can make. I can't do anything about my boss, though. He'll be as last-minute about things as he always is. It's his style.'

'So, one planned change, and now there's your boss and his last-minute reactive management, yes?'

'Yes, and that won't be so easy. I put a lot into my reports when he wants them. I always produce lots of graphs as well as the actual figures themselves.'

'Sounds like you do a lot.' Martin was aware of wondering if Mandy was doing more than she really needed, whether this was an example of her having to justify or prove herself by going further than she actually needed to.

'Yes, I do. Do you think I do too much?' she asked.

Clients often ask direct questions because they want a direct answer, not necessarily because they want to explore why they want the counsellor's opinions or ideas. On some occasions it will be appropriate to explore why they want the counsellor's point of view, but sometimes the client genuinely wants an answer and an attempt to explore the question will generate irritation. A person-centred counsellor might honour both, acknowledging that the client wants an answer and offering the possibility of exploring what meaning she attaches to this need for someone else's view rather than her own.

In this instance, Martin reflects back what he has heard Mandy communicating in terms of her wondering whether she does too much. He might also have taken a different line by saying something like, 'Sounds like you want my opinion and I am wondering what your view is on whether you do too much.'

Martin was aware of not wanting to give an opinion, but rather wanting Mandy to reach her own conclusion for herself. He decided to empathise. 'You feel that you do a lot and you are wondering whether you do too much, yes?'

'I do wonder. Maybe I could cut back on some of the graphs, not too dramatically, but gradually cut back a little and get him used to a little less. Maybe I should talk to the other managers about how they present their figures. I've always just done it my way, wanted to ... here we go again, wanted to show that I could do it. Proving myself again. God, it gets everywhere, doesn't it?'

'Feels like it, huh?'

Mandy shook her head, 'Sure does! Never mind. I've got to get a grip on it all. So, that's two things I can do and they feel realistic. Quite how I'll feel handing over figures with a little less detail than normal, I'm not sure, but I've got to learn to do it that way.'

'Want to explore that or look for something else to change?'

'Another thing that irritates me is the traffic. That wastes a lot of time. It will help having my team come to me more often, but I do have to travel around a lot. If I left earlier some mornings I'm sure I could save time. But if I arrived too early I'd just be waiting there, and while it might be relaxing, I wouldn't be doing anything.' Mandy paused again. She had noticed Martin smiling as she had said that last sentence. 'Oh no, here we go again. Doing again. Why shouldn't I have time to relax? Once I get going I can't stop, and I think I manage to organise my day just to make sure I don't stop. I have to slow down. I need space between appointments. Sometimes we meet up in hotel reception areas, you know? So why not get there early, deliberately, and have a tea or a coffee or something. Give myself time to unwind a bit. I'd probably be in better frame of mind as well.'

'Maybe.'

'OK, so that's three things I can start to do, and I can certainly start changing my travel times and give myself time to relax straight away. I can at least start to reorganise when my team meet up with me. Maybe I should arrange that early on, me coming back after time off would be an opportunity for that. Yes, I'll organise that. They may have to rearrange a few things in their diaries, but I'll get that set up.'

'Seems like you are well on the way to a new style of working and managing your time and your team, and your manager!'

'Yes, I seem to be covering various areas of my work. But it's good. I feel optimistic. These are all realistic strategies. Why I never thought of them before, I suppose I was so into "busy me" that I couldn't see beyond it. Takes something like what has happened to me to stop me in my tracks and cause me to rethink. Even though my instinct has been to want to get back. But the lack of energy and motivation stopped all that. I guess I should be grateful, in a way.'

'Grateful that you lost your motivation and have to take time out. Maybe it was the only way you could stop.'

'I think so. OK. So, these are changes in my working life. I need to relax at home too. I have started that already, I've had to. I've been reading, and actually spending more time just sitting "being" in the garden rather than "doing" in the garden. I know it has been partly because of not feeling very energetic, but maybe I can keep it up, you know? And I have been going out for short walks as well, nothing too strenuous. Maybe I should keep that going as well. That's relaxing. I'm aware that I have developed a different style of walking.'

'A different style?'

'I take my time, I look around more. I stop and just look across the fields and enjoy just being there. I couldn't have done that before. You walked to get somewhere or do something. Now I just dribble along as the feeling takes me, no goals, no time to get back for something. And it is far more satisfying.'

'So this new style of walking leaves you with good feelings, satisfying.'

'And that's it, isn't it? Doing things that satisfy the me that I am, or that I am trying to become. The more I can satisfy the new me, the stronger it will get, and the more normal it will feel.' Mandy stopped, thought for a moment about how she was feeling, and continued. 'I feel really energised by this session today. How are we doing for time? Feels as though we have covered so much and yet it also feels as though time hasn't dragged. Yes, this feels good, and I am really looking forward to putting these ideas into action, and seeing how I feel about it all.'

'We've got a little under ten minutes left. How do you want to use this time?'

Mandy thought for a moment or two. She felt good. She felt positive. She felt as though she was going out to face her first week back with renewed enthusiasm tempered by a sense of feeling able to make choices that would make her working life easier. She was also pleased that she had generally kept her focus during the session without becoming excessively tearful about anything. She felt that this was an achievement.

'I'm pleased that I haven't got too upset or flipped back so much into past experiences. While I've become more aware of the complexity of being me, I also feel more in control. I guess I can move forward now. At the end of the last session we talked about options for more sessions, but the way I feel now, and hopefully will still feel when I see you next week, I think I can move on. That isn't to say I might not need something more in the future, but at the moment I feel satisfied with what I have gained from these sessions. I do feel somehow more complete, as if I have begun to join myself up in some way. That probably sounds weird, but I've begun to appreciate what makes me the person that I am. At least, I can see how the threads of past experience run into my present and affect how I am. But I guess my goal now is to start to weave a new pattern with new threads. The scary thing is having a sense of not knowing what this new pattern will be like. But I do know it will be different, I will be different.'

'So you're feeling more joined up, ready to move on and to weave a new pattern with new threads.'

'Yes, and more complete, more whole somehow. I mean, I'm not sure whether I have completely resolved everything from the past, I'm sure I haven't, but at the moment I simply want to function differently, you know? And if I can achieve that then I will have achieved a lot. Maybe I'll want to achieve more later, I don't know. For now I feel pleased with how I am feeling and I am very aware how different that is to the way I was feeling when I first saw the doctor, and again when I came to see you.' Mandy was sensing a shift in herself and in the nature of her relationship with Martin, though she wasn't sure quite what it was.

It felt to Martin like Mandy was winding up the counselling although they had another session. Maybe she is in a way, kind of ending this part of the process in preparation for moving back to work.

> While endings will have many different meanings and associations for clients, what can easily be overlooked is that a core feature of an ending is that it also represents a transition towards a new beginning. At this point Mandy may be ending in preparation for moving back into work. She may be regarding the final session as almost a one-off to review her beginning back at work rather than a final session of six.

'It feels to me like this is a kind of ending, Mandy. It feels to me as though we have gone through various stages that have brought you to the point at which you feel ready to return to work. So in a sense, there is a completeness in that this goal is now within reach for you. Yet we have a final session next week as well.'

'Maybe that's what I am experiencing. It feels to me like something has ended here today and I do feel somehow liberated in some way.'

'Liberated from?' Martin asked, inviting Mandy to say a little more.

Mandy knew precisely what her response would be. 'My mother.' She sat silently for a few moments reflecting on this. Something in her had moved on, she knew that. She couldn't quite define what it was but something had shifted.

Martin simply reflected back what Mandy had said, 'Liberated from your mother.'

'Sounds awful in a way, but I do feel that way. And I want to acknowledge that she has enabled me to establish a career for myself and to get on in life. She set me up for that, and I am grateful for that.' Mandy suddenly felt herself feeling choked, and tears formed in her eyes and started to trickle down her cheeks. 'And I won't be able to thank her now.'

'You'd like to thank her. . . .' Martin didn't complete his reflection, he wanted to leave the emphasis on the *wanting* to thank her rather than the *what* to be thanked about.

Mandy nodded, and reached for a tissue. She felt a burning feeling in her throat as the tears continued to roll down her face. 'I just want to say thank you. I know I've got other feelings about being conditioned into being busy, but I am grateful as well.' The tears continued to escape from her eyes as Mandy buried her face in her hands. 'You did your best for me, mum, I know you did. I know you loved me really, but it was so hard to feel it.' The burning in her throat became more intense and the tears got heavier. She began to sob more loudly. 'I love you mum, I love you so much, and I miss you so. Oh God, I miss you. I wish you were here. I wish we could spend time together, you and me, doing whatever.' Mandy stopped speaking but the tears continued to flow. She felt unable to stop them; she didn't want them to stop. She felt like they were flowing straight from her heart, hot and wet and full of hurt and sadness.

Martin had noticed that time had passed and that the session should end, however he had no further client that day and felt it appropriate to let the session run on.

When is it appropriate to overrun a session and what consideration should inform the decision? In this instance, the client has been suddenly overwhelmed by feelings. It seems unlikely that she had much control over them. She would have been carrying a sense of her loss and her upset, but she had chosen a different focus for this session. Martin does not have a client after her so he hasn't got to consider his commitment to the next person. He may wish to reflect on whether Mandy has introduced these feelings deliberately at the end in order to extend the session – perhaps an expression of her wanting more time. Or, as in this case, it could simply be that a focus in the session which could have happened at any time, simply occurred near the end and it enabled Mandy to connect with feelings that were probably near the surface anyway, and just needed the right therapeutic moment to come out.

These feelings had not been planned to arise at this time. Mandy needed this release, needed to own her feelings for her mother. So he said nothing about the time and maintained his empathic focus on Mandy. He really felt for her as she sat there sobbing, lost in the ocean of feelings that had rushed in upon her. He didn't say anything, choosing to sit and remain attentive to Mandy, and allow himself to feel warmth and caring for her as a person in pain, a human being like himself that had the capacity to experience the emotions of loss with all the intensity.... His train of thought was interrupted. Mandy was speaking again.

'Why did she have to leave me? I feel alone without her. I know she didn't go on purpose, but it hurts so much. I don't like these feelings. They feel so deep.' Her breathing had become short and sharp, gulping air in through her mouth and letting it back out with a kind of shudder. She swallowed but could not stop the tears.

'Here, have another tissue,' Martin said softly, as he reached across. Mandy took it and blew her nose. But the tears continued.

'Oh God.' She swallowed again. 'Oh God.' Mandy could feel a cold sensation in her body and she shuddered. She shook her head and began to take her hands away, looking up into Martin's eyes. Her mascara was now smudged around her eyes and down her cheeks. Her eyes were very red. The tears had not abated. She blinked, and swallowed again. Taking a deep breath, she yawned. 'Oh, sorry.' She took another deep breath, which triggered another yawn. 'I feel suddenly very tired. Just now I was feeling so energised and now I feel all limp.' Mandy breathed in deeply and breathed out with a long sigh. 'I wasn't expecting any of that. But it must have been in me needing to come out.' She was beginning to feel a little clearer now but still felt as though all the energy had been drained out of her.

Martin nodded, 'Yeah,' he said gently.

'What time is it? I ought to be going.' Mandy looked anxiously at Martin and towards the clock on the wall.

'It's OK, take the time that you need. I'm not seeing anyone else so just,' he nodded, 'just take your time.'

'Thanks. I think I'll need a few moments to get myself together. I'd almost suggested heading off when you asked what I wanted to do with the last ten minutes. I think I'm glad that I didn't. Why are emotions so draining? I feel really wobbly, really wobbly.'

Martin had decided not to continue overdoing the empathy, but to give Mandy the space she needed to slowly bring herself back together. 'You may need to have a stretch, yawn a few more times, get yourself back into your body a bit.'

Mandy stretched and promptly broke into an enormous yawn, bringing her hands quickly in front of her mouth and blinking with an astonished look in her eyes. She took in another breath deeply before letting it out slowly. She picked up the glass of water and drank deeply. 'That's better. Beginning to feel a little less wobbly now. I think I'm OK to head off now. Same time next week?'

'Yes. Before you head out you might like to fix your mascara though.'

'Oh God, yes, is it that bad?' Mandy got out her mirror. 'Oh yes, it is that bad. Thanks.' She wiped off the smudges and thanked Martin again for reminding her.

'No problem. Good luck with work.'

'Oh, yes. That seems ages ago we were talking about that. Those feelings were so intense. They just took over, totally. There was nothing else, just those feelings. My throat is still burning. I'll get some more water from the machine outside before I go. I'll see you next week and let you know how I got on. Thanks again.' Mandy got up and left the counselling room, feeling a mixture of relief and unsteadiness. It hadn't been comfortable but she did feel as though she had released some strong, pent-up feelings. She knew she still felt upset, but it felt more tolerable now. In fact, she kind of felt glad she felt upset. It somehow felt right. Yes, she was grateful to her mother. And yes, there were other feelings around as well going back to those early years, but for now the feelings of gratitude and loss were uppermost.

Martin waited a minute or two and then went out himself for some water. He also felt as though he had been hit by a tidal wave of feelings. Probably the more so because he hadn't been expecting it. One moment it seemed that the session had virtually ended and then, whoosh, the tears had started flowing. He needed a few minutes to get himself back into focus as well. He decided to make himself a cup of tea. By the time he returned to the counselling room with it he was beginning to feel his focus coming back. He sat down to reflect on the session. It had felt good. A lot of positive ideas had come out of it and Mandy had made a lot of assertive decisions about the changes she wanted to make at work. He felt good that they had been her ideas as well.

He was also pleased that Mandy had got in touch with her feelings of loss towards her mother, and the gratitude as well. Bereavement isn't only about acknowledging losses but also allowing the things that one was grateful for to be celebrated. Mandy had a lot of good reasons to have real mixed feelings about her mother. How she would be affected by this release, only time would tell. But it had felt healthy and natural, spontaneous and unforced. Mandy's own process had taken her into those feelings and he firmly believed in trusting that process. OK, so he had overrun the session, and maybe it might have been different had there been another client waiting, or maybe not. He felt that his duty was towards the client he was with and helping to ensure that she was feeling ready to leave. Sometimes the next client had to wait. No doubt there would be many different views about this but in the context of that afternoon he felt comfortable with his decision to allow Mandy more time.

Client case notes

Client arrived more confident. Expressed anger, frustration, determination. Discussed impact of her mother's style of working on her and explored further her tendency to be busy and her need to justify herself as being good enough. Plans to return to work next week. Discussed changes she wants to make to reduce stress. Tearful release of feelings towards her mother as she expressed gratitude towards her for doing her best.

Points for discussion/action

- Discuss the nature of endings from the standpoint that an ending marks the start of a transition towards a new beginning.
- If you felt emotionally affected by a client such that you found yourself unable to hold a clear focus for your next client, what steps would you take?
- Was it appropriate to overrun the session? In what circumstances would you allow this? How would you have handled it if another client had been due?
- How would you feel if Mandy did not attend her final session, and that Martin's sense of Mandy's ending was accurate? How would you react and what would you do, and why?
- Critically evaluate the counselling session.
- Make your own clinical notes of this session.

'I haven't so much to say about Mandy today, Anne. I have only seen her for one appointment since I last saw you as she was unwell one week. Mind you, the session that we did have was a bit of a roller-coaster ride. Well, it was right at the end.'

'So it got a bit, what, intense?' Anne replied, wanting to clarify a little more what it had felt like.

'Very intense. Suddenly Mandy started grieving heavily for her mother, completely out of the blue. I wasn't expecting it. The session had not been particularly emotional, but just as we were into the final ten minutes and the session seemed to be winding down, well, it took me by surprise.'

'Mhmm. Really took you by surprise.'

'Yeah. Up until then the session had largely focused on what changes she was going to make when she returned to work.'

Anne was aware of frowning slightly, she had the idea that Mandy wasn't heading back to work just yet, somehow she had got the idea that she was going to be off for a while. She voiced her thoughts. 'I was thinking Mandy was going to be off work longer. Did I get that wrong?'

'No, I was expecting her to be off work, in fact the GP had dropped in on the day that Mandy did not attend and wanted to know how she was getting on. I didn't disclose much, but we did talk about how much time she might need to get ready to return to work, and both felt it would take a while. Anyway, the next time Mandy saw Dr Hill she had persuaded her that she was ready to go back to work, and that was that. Mandy goes back next week, and I see her for her last session next week.' Martin was aware of his own unease coming back over all of this, although he couldn't really say why. It just seemed too quick, somehow, given the depth of the conditions of worth that Mandy had experienced as a child when she was fostered out and the impact of her mother with her focus on work and being busy.

'You don't look too comfortable about it, Martin.' Anne was noticing that Martin didn't seem too relaxed, he looked a bit tense as he had been talking.

'I'm not, but I can't really be specific about it. But I just sense that Mandy is hoping to have changed around a pattern that has been stuck for life in, what, five sessions. And I have my doubts. But I also have to say that I hope she has.

Maybe she has made enough change in herself to sustain a fresh approach to working and her lifestyle generally. I really hope that she has if that is what she wants. But I know I'm not sure.'

Anne nodded. She was thinking about how a limited period of counselling could leave counsellors feeling that the work had only really begun. It could mean a sense of incompleteness and lack of a sense of fulfilment in the counselling process. Yet forced closure on the counselling relationship did not mean that the client stopped working on the issues. The client's growth process would continue and often the hard part for a counsellor lay in accepting that they would only travel part of the journey with their client, and that they had to let go and trust that they had helped the client become more self-aware and able to choose to be a way that satisfied them. 'So, not sure whether the changes she is planning can be sustained and built upon. To you it feels as though five sessions is too short.'

Martin sat thinking for a minute. Yes, he thought, I know what it is. He voiced his thoughts. 'It's the falseness of it all that is troubling me.'

Anne was unsure what Martin meant. 'Can you tell me more?'

'Mandy is going back now partly because she wants to try it and still have a session to talk it through with me. I don't think she would be choosing to go back if the counselling was ongoing. I have a sense, and I could be wrong because I don't know what Mandy is thinking or feeling about this, it is an assumption. But I think that Mandy is wanting to use our last session as a kind of safety net because she isn't sure either. I'm sure she wants to feel she will be able to come back and say how well she has done and to be able to end the counselling on a really positive and encouraging note. But there is a risk of it not being quite like that, and maybe part of her recognises this and also sees that final session as a support if things go wrong, or don't work out as she is planning.'

'I'm struck by the fact that she doesn't have a lot of time at work anyway – what, three days before she sees you? Not much time to really know how she is coping and making changes.'

'Yeah. But I am still aware that these are our thoughts, and I don't know what is motivating Mandy to go back now, other than she did emphasise the idea of going back and having that final session afterwards. That seemed to be coming across to me as the main reason. She talked of having more energy but..., I don't know. I'm concerned. I felt that in the session but didn't voice it. I really didn't want to undermine her. She could be right. She may have done enough, but I know I'm not convinced.'

Anne was reflecting on whether to hold Martin with his concerns and allow him to explore them, or shift to what he felt he needed to do about his concern. She chose the former, that being where Martin actually was in himself at this time. 'Is she going back too soon and has the fact of there being only the one session left encouraged her to return to work sooner rather than later? You don't know, you're concerned.'

'Yeah, I am. But I don't know whether to say anything.' Martin thought for a moment and realised, of course, that he couldn't plan to say anything as he didn't know what Mandy would experience in those first three days back at work. He felt he would know what to say when they met up next week, but what he could sense nagging at him now was why he hadn't said anything in the session. 'Maybe I should have said something in the session, Anne. Maybe I should have trusted myself in what I was experiencing, and Mandy to hear it as a concern rather than as a questioning of her decision.'

> Martin's uneasiness and lack of trust (of himself and Mandy) has obstructed his ability to be transparent. This is crucial. The ability of the person-centred therapist to be congruent plays an important part in creating the therapeutic climate within which the client can undergo constructive personality change.

'Never any guarantees how a client will hear something that you say, but your wonder now is whether you should have said something. You lost your transparency.'

'I did. I can see it now. I didn't want to undermine Mandy.' Martin thought for a moment and he began to feel he was getting some clarity about what was happening. 'You know, it seems as though it isn't only Mandy who has adjusted to making what feels like for her the best use of the six sessions. So have I.'

'So you feel that you have both in some way adjusted to the time frame that you have.'

'Yes. I mean, I was holding back because I wanted Mandy to leave after her last session with the confidence that she came with, and I didn't want to risk undermining that. Had we had more sessions I think I would have said something, in fact, I'm sure I would. But it is as though it became harder for me to be congruent because I was thinking this way.'

'Makes short-term work quite challenging to our approach where the counsellor's ability to be congruent is such an important element in the therapeutic work.'

'Yes,' Martin replied, 'it does, but that is no excuse. However long I have with a client, I need to bring my authentic self into that therapeutic space. I haven't been as helpful to Mandy as I could have been.' Martin reflected for a moment and he was aware of feeling somewhat pissed off with himself. He continued, 'Makes me feel somewhat pissed off with myself, yet it feels like the moment has passed now. Whether I say anything next session will depend on what transpires in the session. But there were things I could have said last session, I'm sure.'

'So your sense is that you weren't helpful to Mandy but that the moment may have passed. What might you have said?' Anne was feeling that it could be helpful for Martin to bring into words whatever was on his mind, if only to release it.

Martin thought back to the session. How had it gone? What had Mandy being saying, and what had he been feeling? 'I remember my unease when Mandy said she was going back. I said something like, "So, going back next week then," and I remember trying to say it in a kind of bland sort of way, not wanting to sound doubting of the wisdom of it, and yet not sounding totally devoid of feeling. It felt wrong somehow, I just wasn't expressing what I was feeling and thinking. It wasn't a congruent response. It was incongruent. But I justified it to myself by deciding to maintain my empathy on Mandy. But ... I don't think I made the right choice, Anne. It troubles me.'

'Troubled by your incongruence in that moment,' Anne replied, seeking to hold the focus on Martin's discomfort.

'I didn't want to cause her to feel I didn't support her in her decision.'

'Mhmm.' Anne could feel herself wanting to know why, wanting to clarify what this was about. 'I feel I really want to ask "why?" '

Martin sighed, 'I don't know. I could have said something like, "You're really sure it is time to go back?" but even then I can feel myself thinking, yes, but I'd have to say it in a way that won't upset her or direct her away from her own decision.'

'Not directing her away is an appropriate reason, but not upsetting her?' Anne was aware of feeling concerned.

Clients have a right to feel how they need to feel. Martin would not be deliberately seeking to cause upset, he would be being transparent as to his genuine concerns. How the client then reacts is according to her needs. What has happened is that Mandy has effectively been directed away from the opportunity to explore whatever might be present for her if she engaged with the thought that she could be going back too soon.

'I think I'm struggling a bit with theory here. I mean, I don't want to be directive and I don't want to question her own internal process of evaluating her situation and formulating a response that is realistic to her. God, that sounds a mouthful. But I want to feel able to be authentically me, and I wasn't.' Martin sat back in his chair. 'I got pushed out of my congruence, Anne, I can see that. I got blocked, and I know the block was coming from me. I don't believe that the client made me behave this way. I made a choice, and I am damn sure it wasn't the right one, or let's say the most therapeutically helpful. Dammit, I'm supposed to be authentic with my clients, I owe them that at the very least.'

Anne had noticed that Martin had raised his voice and looked more than a little heated. 'You sound pretty fired up about all this, Martin.'

Martin felt the smile spread across his face spontaneously. 'You know, I said something about being fired up to Mandy in that session. What was it? Yeah, she'd been talking about going back to work and her drive to be busy, and then said something about having a bit of energy and immediately feeling she had to go back to work. That's right, she had begun to question herself about going back to work. Oh, yes, and there had been a discussion around whether her drive to be busy was learned from her mother or something more genetic and deep-seated, and did that mean she was powerless to change. Anyway, she got very fired up, angry, not wanting to make the same mistake of overdoing it, wanting to be in control. I remember she said she was quite angry with herself.'

'Angry with herself.'

'And frustrated as well. She went on to talk about feeling like she had got into this damn rut, and that she had to get out of it and learn to stay out of it. She was very determined and I remember matching her tone of voice. Then she suddenly went quieter, having got a sense of the immensity of the changes before her. But then she got back into that stronger part and affirmed how she had to change, that she had to move on and make choices that kept her away from that busy, busy, busy pattern.'

'You know, there's a word that I haven't heard you use but it is very present for me as I hear you speaking, Martin. *Desperation*. It all sounds very desperate.'

'Yes.' Martin thought for a moment, yes, that really did sum it up, and he suddenly became aware of the tension in his own body. He had sat forward again in his chair and his back had tightened up. He sat back again. 'It's leaving me with a lot of tension, I know that.'

Anne decided to stay with this, although she was still carrying concern from earlier, linked to how Martin, while saying he was non-directive, had unwittingly directed Mandy away from focusing on the concerns that were present about her going back too soon. But for now she wanted to stay with Martin, whose body seemed to be telling him something that he needed to pay attention to insofar as his own process was concerned. 'You're feeling physically tense.'

'I am, right across my back and shoulders.'

'What does it feel like?'

'Like a heavy weight making the top of my shoulders sore, but also my back, just below the area beneath my shoulder blades.' He raised his shoulders and bent forward a little, trying to ease the knot that was present in his back. He twisted one shoulder up, then the other. 'Gee, it's tight.'

'Given how you are experiencing this tightness, Martin, can you imagine what would cause it in real life?'

'What do you mean?'

'Well, what might you have to be doing, physically, to get the sensation of tension and tightness you are experiencing?'

Martin thought about it. 'Certainly some kind of weight across the shoulders, but not just that. Maybe if I was pushing something as well. Yes, that's it. If I was pushing something. But no, my arms aren't tense. It's in my shoulders and back.' He thought about it more and tried to imagine what posture he would need to be in to experience this tightness. 'Got it! You know those images you see of oxen pulling a plough, or something like that, with the harness thing round their necks and over their shoulders? That's it. Beast of burden. It feels like a heavy weight I'm dragging behind me, but I'm doing it by pushing with my shoulders. What's that all about?' Martin stretched and yawned, trying to ease the tightness a little.

'Tired of it?' Anne responded quickly to the yawn.

'Yeah. I want to get out of it and feel free.'

'You want to feel free.'

'Yes, I sure do. God, yes.'

Anne was aware of Mandy again. 'OK, so what meaning does it have in relation to Mandy, and your relationship with her?'

'I guess Mandy must feel as though she has realised for the first time in her life
   that she is dragging this weight around, the way of being that she learned earlier in her life, and has now tasted something of what it is like to be free of it, or
   at least to have a little less weight. And I guess she wants more of that freedom.
   Must be a very powerful experience. You know, the thought has just struck me
   that I wasn't aware of feeling so stiff until I suddenly became aware of it. I know
   that sounds daft, but that's how it is, isn't it? We aren't aware of things until
   suddenly we are. Mandy wasn't aware of how she has been in terms of having
   learned it from her mother until she suddenly recognised it.' Martin stopped
   and thought for a moment. 'But how on earth did it all get into my body?'
'Good question. How on earth did it get into your body?'
Martin thought about it. He could see two possibilities. 'Well, either I have something that I feel the same way about and it has triggered that off for me in some
   way, making me more aware of feeling burdened, or by focusing on what is
   happening for Mandy, something about her has got into me. But then, I don't
   think anything could affect me like this unless there was already something
   there for it to hook into or resonate with in some way.'
'OK, so you suspect there is something in you that feels burdensome which in
   some way may, or may not, have a connection with what Mandy is experiencing.' Anne had an idea as to what it might be, but she wanted Martin to make
   his own connection. She might be wrong anyway, but she kind of felt that she
   was right, that it was to do with the burden of working in a contained, six-
   session way. She asked a direct question: 'What do you find burdensome, or constraining?' She added 'constraining' as it just sounded right to say it somehow.
'I don't know about burdensome but constraining immediately brings to mind
   this whole question of working to six sessions.' Martin stopped and an image
   came to mind. He smiled.
'Yes,' Anne replied, 'something's made you smile.'
'Yes, well I could see myself as the oxen and what I am pushing against is the six-
   session limit. I'm not dragging anything, I'm pushing it with my shoulders but
   I'm also strapped to it.' He sighed and felt himself relax a little. 'That's it, isn't it?
   It's me and the limitation of six sessions, and wanting to push that boundary
   but I can't. And of course it is having an impact on Mandy, and I guess it has
   heightened in me that sense of the weight of it all. OK, I need to reflect on this
   some more. I need to make my peace with this time limited way of working.
   I need to change my attitude. Well, maybe I need to understand my attitude
   more.' Martin looked at the clock.
'So, you sense a need for greater understanding of your attitude towards this way
   of working. Is there anything else you want to explore on this theme, Martin?'
'No. I've spent much more time than I planned talking about Mandy, but it
   has been really useful. And it has certainly given me something to think
   about. I haven't been owning my true feelings about working this way, have I?
   I mean, I knew I wasn't at ease with it, but it runs deeper than that. I need to
   think more about it and reflect on whether there are other aspects to me that
   feed into it. Seems like it could be an issue to explore in personal therapy, or
   in the group of counsellors that I meet up with who also work in primary

healthcare. I think I'll start with the group, we meet up again in two weeks, and I'll raise the issue there. See what happens. And I may take it to therapy, and I may bring it back here as well.'

At what point does an issue become a factor for personal therapy rather than supervision? I do not believe in rigidity regarding this. There is surely something of an overlap. Where a reaction from a counsellor can be dealt with in supervision without it impacting on the need to spend time on other work, then that seems appropriate. However, where an issue comes up again and again then clearly it has not been resolved and personal therapy is the place to take this.

Person-centred supervision is likely to place a lot of emphasis on the counsellor's experience of working with the client, and the nature of the relationship that they are building. It is therefore likely that this supervision will involve more supervisee content. There will be those areas of experiencing within the supervisee that are pertinent to the therapeutic relationship that will be dealt with in supervision. However, there will also be content and reaction that are clearly rooted in the supervisee's own incongruence within his structure of self that makes it difficult for him to be able to empathically sense and reflect what the client is seeking to communicate. Where this cannot be resolved in supervision then personal therapy will be required.

'Seems like you want to get to the bottom of it and, yes, maybe you need some time to reflect on it, discuss it with others, but bring it back here as well because clearly it could be having an impact on your work with other clients.' Anne was aware that she hadn't forgotten about the issue of why Martin had not been authentic towards Mandy when she was talking of going back to work. 'We're still left with the issue of why you didn't voice your unease to Mandy, though.'

'Yes, I'd forgotten that. You're good at holding on to issues and bringing them back. OK. I need to think about this a moment and get back into that focus.' A thought struck him almost immediately. 'I think I have a sense of what it was, and talking about what we have just been addressing I think has loosened it up for me. I think it is something to do with wanting to feel that Mandy has moved on within the six sessions, and not wanting to say anything that would undermine that. I think the six-session limit is encouraging me to want my clients to reach their goal, and maybe it is this that blocked me from voicing my unease. Maybe I didn't want her to start doubting what she had planned to do. I wanted to keep her process nicely fitting within the six-session box. Does that make sense? It does to me, and that's scary because it is changing how I work. And I'm not sure about that.'

'So you think that the boundary of six sessions affected whether you were able to be authentic with your client, fearing that she might not do as well, or at least leave the final session with unmet needs.'

'Yes, and I know that it is ridiculous in a sense. I have to trust the client's own process and their recognition that they have six sessions and that is the time-scale that they work to. And I can see that Mandy is doing this as well in terms of her timing to go back to work. Seems like she has adjusted to it and I'm struggling with it. I've got to get clarity on this, Anne, and think about my own practice in this context. I know that I can apply a person-centred approach to any time period. Wasn't Carl Rogers asked once what he would do if he had only ten minutes with a client and replied he would offer them ten minutes of therapy!' Martin was not best pleased with himself, as he really had a clear sense that he had not adjusted to six-session working and that he needed to resolve it. But at least it did help him make sense of his lack of authenticity.

'Yes, we have to work within the limits of what is available, and so long as it is clear and visible to the client then we must trust that they will use that time in whatever way their own actualising tendency urges them. And yes, there will be times when it will not be enough and we have to then refer on.'

'Yes. I guess I'm accustomed to working with people through a whole therapeutic process and I get frustrated if I feel I can only go part of the distance because of external factors that I have no control over.' Martin looked at the time. 'I really do need to spend a little time on other clients, Anne. I will give more thought to all of this, but I would like to move on.'

'I hear you say you want to move on, but there is still something nagging at me and I need to bring us back to it. You mentioned earlier that mentioning your concerns would have to be done in a way that won't upset her or direct her away from her own decision. "Won't upset her" does not feel comfortable. We are not there to direct or protect clients from their discomfort, you know that, so what was that about?'

Martin smiled, 'I love the way that you remain open to your feelings and express them. It's exactly what I was struggling with.'

'I was aware that it might be tempting not to say anything as we had moved on, but it remained present, and I was aware of the risk of parallel processing.' Anne was aware that she didn't want the focus to slide back to theory and decided to make it clear and sharp. 'So, you didn't want to upset Mandy.'

An example of parallel processing is where some pattern of behaviour in the counsellor–client relationship gets lived out in the supervisor–supervisee relationship. In this case, Martin's inability to voice his authentic concerns and be transparent to his client could have been paralleled by Anne not mentioning her concerns regarding Martin saying he didn't want to upset his client. These kinds of dynamics have to be watched for. The supervisor's heightened self-awareness and congruence provides the means whereby she can sense whether she is acting out of character. Sometimes it goes unnoticed in the session, but the supervisor may then carry this process into her supervision and it is hoped that it will be recognised then.

'No, I didn't, but I'm really not sure why. Was I protecting her? Was I wanting her to succeed and felt I might. . . ,' Martin had a sudden thought. 'I'm wondering whether I felt she had had enough upset over those sessions. But that's ridiculous. I know that isn't how I feel about this work, but there is something about Mandy, isn't there. But I don't know what it is. Of course I can't go around stopping my clients getting upset. That really is a personal therapy issue, Anne. My sense is that this is only a Mandy-oriented reaction on my part, but I need to talk this through and get into my own experiencing on this. I think that my now heightened awareness of it is going to help me offset it if it comes up again in our final session. But I do want to get to grips with this and if there is a block in me then I have to find out what it is and explore it. I do think it is linked to my work with Mandy, though.' Martin sat and ran images of his other clients in front of him, trying to discern whether he sensed he had in any way been blocking them from being upset. It just didn't ring true as he thought of recent sessions with these clients. 'I'm just thinking about my other clients, but I can't see anything to indicate I'm not letting them get upset. If anything, it feels the opposite! Personal therapy and I'll also keep you informed of what I get from it, Anne. Do you think that's the best way forward?'

Anne felt at ease with this. The tension she had been carrying around this issue had lifted. She was glad she had voiced it and that Martin had responded positively. He could have been defensive, but one strength of Martin's that she admired was his commitment to his ongoing personal development so that he could be fully and authentically present within the therapeutic relationship. 'That feels OK, Martin, but I'd be interested to know what you find out as it would be useful for me to be mindful of in future supervision sessions.'

'No problem, I can appreciate that. So, shall we move on?

After the supervision session, and on his journey home, Martin was thinking about how he really needed to trust Mandy's own actualising tendency, that she was making choices that, given the context, were most reasonable and which, for her, minimised the risk of anxiety and discomfort. Yes, there was a lot of hurt associated with her past, and it had left her with particular personality traits that she now had mixed feelings about. Yet she was an adult and capable of making her own decisions. As he pondered on this Martin was aware that he was beginning to feel somehow uneasy about something. What had triggered it off? He pulled the car over into a lay-by. He just sensed that something important was moving around on the edge of his awareness, but he couldn't quite grab hold of it.

The words that started to come back to him more forcibly were those he had just been thinking about, 'she was an adult and capable of making her own decisions'. Of course he knew that. She was a successful career woman, making decisions and choices all the time and, OK, so she had become overwhelmed, but she was certainly capable of making decisions. He recognised that the therapeutic process of counselling had helped her to rethink her attitude towards work and to plan changes. Yet he was still uneasy.

As he was sitting there trying to make sense of it he realised that in fact his mind had begun to go blank, he was just sitting, staring out of the window but without really taking anything in. Suddenly the words from that earlier session came forcibly to mind. He heard Mandy saying them, 'please don't make me'. He felt the goosebumps break out over his arms and up his neck. And he felt tears in his eyes and a lump in his throat. He closed his eyes, trying to stay with the feelings that were beginning to clarify inside himself. Fear. Fear of the unknown. Loneliness. The sense of not being heard. Abandonment. Powerlessness. All the feelings that a four-year-old might experience when made to do something she did not want to do, or lose something that was precious and familiar. The feelings began to subside and Martin took a deep breath and blinked, seeking to bring himself back to focus yet also wanting to honour the presence of what he was feeling.

My God, he thought, I'm still carrying that and it is very much present. He then began to wonder what effect it may have been having on his work with Mandy. It suddenly came to him that he had not really been fully relating to her as an adult. He couldn't have been, with this strength of feeling present towards her as a little girl. Had he been trying to protect her in some way? Oh-oh, he was filled with a disturbing thought. She's just about young enough to have been my daughter. Was I wanting to offer her more sessions because I wanted to protect her and support her? Was I allowing a kind of fathering impulse to get into the sessions? He was aware that he was now very much back in his head, trying to think back. Had that been why he had felt so uneasy at not voicing his concern? Was it more than feeling time was limited?

He continued to reflect on this insight and didn't reach any firm conclusion. But he acknowledged to himself that he needed to be aware that perhaps he was not fully engaging in an adult-to-adult relationship in the counselling, or at least, he was at risk of slipping away from it. He asked himself whether he really thought of Mandy the adult as a daughter figure, and the more he thought about it, the more that didn't feel how it was. No, it was her as the four-year-old that was making the impact, but could that still have affected him when he was with her and she was not expressing that aspect of herself?

He made a mental note to take that back to supervision. But he knew he wanted to clear this in personal therapy. It had hooked into him and that meant there was something within himself that was sensitive to this area of experiencing. He did not believe feelings were transferred into him for no reason, but rather that they had a powerful impact because there was something about himself that resonated to the feeling tone of the client. He had to look at himself. If he had sensitivities that he was not aware of but which were affecting his behaviour, then he was being incongruent. And that was not good enough. He was aware that Mandy only had one more session, but she might come back for more and he needed to develop clarity as to the true origin and nature of his feelings. OK, time to head off. He sat up a little more upright in the seat, turned the key in the ignition and turned back on to the road.

Clients can and do have a powerful impact on counsellors and sometimes the full impact is not recognised at the time, but can make an impression later. Martin clearly needs to work this through. It is OK to be affected by clients, in fact, some would argue it is necessary to be an effective therapist. But the counsellor needs to be aware that he is affected and how. Otherwise, congruence is lost and behaviours within the therapeutic setting may emerge that are at the very least unhelpful and at worse damaging to the client. Martin may be advised to at least discuss this with Anne on the phone before he sees Mandy again.

Points for discussion

- If you had been Martin, would you have responded to Anne differently, and if so, how?
- Discuss what kind of issues you might be particularly sensitive to and are at risk of being incongruent around.
- What issues do you experience in yourself regarding working in a time limited way?
- Critically evaluate Anne's work in this session and whether you feel the issues that needed to be addressed were addressed.
- Is this a situation in which Martin should talk through with Anne his experience in the lay-by before he next sees Mandy?

SESSION 7

Martin did phone Anne and spent time talking through the feelings he had
become aware of as being present within him during his lay-by experience.
He was grateful for this. It had left him feeling more able to hold an adult focus
with Mandy. He felt that the fact this was to be the last session required
him to be fully present as an adult with her. He recognised that he had been
affected by that earlier session but somehow that had lifted. He had expressed
a lot of emotion over the phone and it had made a difference. He somehow felt
lighter as he waited as the clock ticked towards the start time of the counselling session.

Mandy was sitting in the waiting room. She had arrived a few minutes early. She
was quite glad to be able to just sit there, thumbing through the magazines.
None of them was particularly interesting, but they kind of helped her to
switch off. It had been a hectic few days and she was glad she had this counselling appointment. It wasn't that she was not coping, she simply felt glad to
have a bit of time to reflect on how things were going. She was feeling quite
tired as well.

She saw Martin come out and she got up and followed him to the counselling
room. She sat down and waited. She knew she had things to say, but she had
actually got quite relaxed sitting out there and still felt kind of lethargic. She
heard Martin begin to speak.

'So, how do you want to use today's session, your final one of the six.'

Mandy thought about it. 'I'm not sure. I mean, I have things to talk about but
right at the moment I'm just feeling very lethargic. I haven't felt this way all
week, well not at work, and actually not that much in the evenings. But sitting
out there just now, I guess I got too comfortable and with the music playing
in the background, I guess I just drifted.' She smiled. 'And I actually feel OK
about it too! I really think I am accepting just *being*, I don't know, less frenetic.
I mean, it does feel a little strange if I really think about it, but otherwise I
think I am learning to. . . , well, to just be.' Mandy thought for a moment, there
was something not quite right about that. 'No, I don't want to say *just* be, I want
to say *be*. *Just* seems to weaken it and I am realising that being is not a weakness,
it is a strength.'

Martin nodded. 'So, finding it feels OK to *be* and feeling lethargic towards say-ing anything.'

'That's right.' Mandy paused. She kind of felt she ought to say something about how the week had gone since returning to work Monday morning. Just as she was about to start she suddenly remembered again how the last session had ended. 'You know, the tears, my tears, at the end of the last session really did shift something. I didn't feel too sure when I left, felt rather fragile. But that gradually passed as the day wore on. I did a bit of shopping and visited a friend in the evening. We talked about this and that, and it suddenly struck me as I was talking to her how relaxed I felt. I told her this and she said that she had noticed that I didn't seem to be on edge, "like you usually are". I asked Jo, my friend, if it had been that obvious, and she said that she had accepted it as being the way that I was. But she hadn't really thought about it much until she saw the contrast in me that evening. Said I just looked more relaxed, somehow, more easy going. It felt really, really good hearing her tell me that. I actually reached out and gave her a hug, and that really wasn't me. Took Jo by surprise as well! But it felt really good.' Mandy suddenly went quiet, and felt embarrassed. 'I'm talking a lot, aren't I?'

Martin felt pleased and was struck by the memory that in an earlier session Mandy had said something about talking too much and had seemed to sud-denly go very self-conscious. He tried to remember back to the occasion, but couldn't connect with it. He brought himself back to the present. 'You look a bit embarrassed by it. But I really feel good myself that you have not only felt more relaxed but have had positive feedback from a friend.' He felt that he was being empathic in acknowledging what he had heard Mandy tell him and he had made visible what he was experiencing as well.

This kind of response is powerful. It expresses empathy, warm acceptance of what the client has said and a congruent expression of what the counsellor is experiencing.

'It's not easy talking about yourself, or at least, I seem to find it difficult to own up to having had positive things said about me.'

'So, feeling embarrassed is more about being able to talk about the positive feed-back from others than simply talking about yourself?'

'Yes, though I'm not sure if it is so much embarrassment as just feeling, you know, kind of uncomfortable.'

Martin nodded, 'Uncomfortable....' Martin nodded again, he was aware of puzzling as to whether Mandy was saying it was the feeling positive, receiving positive feedback, or talking about positive feedback that made her uncomfor-table. He realised that he was unclear and decided he needed to say a little more. 'I need to check out because I am unclear. Is it the feeling positive that is uncomfortable, or the receiving of positive feedback, or the talking about it?'

When a counsellor is in doubt about something it is helpful to clarify it then and there. Saves possible confusion later and it is another example of a congruent response. However, such a question would not be appropriate if it was simply rooted in idle curiosity. The need to know has to be recognised as having therapeutic value, enabling the counsellor to empathically appreciate what is present for the client.

Mandy thought for a moment. She had been tempted to just say 'talking about it', but she had held back because she could remember feeling uncomfortable when Jo had said how relaxed she seemed. Was uncomfortable too strong a word, though? She certainly felt uncomfortable talking about it, but when Jo had said she looked relaxed it had been more that she didn't quite know what to do or say. In fact, she remembered her whole body sort of didn't quite know what to do with itself. Oh dear, she thought, how do I describe all this. She heard Martin say, 'You're giving it a lot of thought.'

'Yes, because I think I'm feeling different things. I did feel uncomfortable talking about it, but receiving it I felt, well, I don't know if I'd say it was uncomfortable, it just kind of felt, well, kind of. . . ,' Mandy wasn't sure what to say, so she finally said, 'kind of weird.'

That, thought Martin, could mean a number of things. He just reflected back the word with a hint of questioning in his voice. 'Weird?'

'Yes, kind of confused me, didn't know what to say or do, you know. Just, I don't know, just weird I guess.'

'Kind of confused, not knowing what to say or do, just kind of weird.' That, Martin thought, would probably look really odd if someone read a transcript of this session, but it had felt right to just reflect it back and let Mandy know he was with her. He was aware that as he spoke he was frowning slightly.

This kind of empathic response is not something you would hear in ordinary conversation, but then counselling is *not* ordinary conversation.

'You can look confused, so am I!' Mandy replied, having noticed the frown and taking it to mean that Martin wasn't sure what she was talking about. It actually felt good to know he was confused, it kind of validated her confusion, made it feel a little easier to accept somehow. 'Good to know I'm not alone,' she added with a smile.

Martin smiled but was also aware that the focus had shifted very rapidly from something uncomfortable to something humorous. He realised that this might be what some would call a defence. He saw it as a positive action to preserve a sense of wellbeing.

From a person-centred perspective, 'defences' are behaviours that emerge from the person's structure of self in response to experiences that threaten to expose discomfort or hurt. This is a natural and healthy reaction. Defences have a purpose and the client in a person-centred relationship is trusted to address these defences as and when she feels ready and able. Pushing a client to drop her defences is not a feature of person-centred counselling. It can leave her exposed and vulnerable beyond what her own process of being can sustain. The person-centred counsellor trusts the client's organismic self to know what is sustainable. The offering of the warmth of unconditional positive regard and empathy allows the client to feel safe enough to expose defences.

Also, anything that threatens the client's structure of self is likely to be defended against in order to preserve that out of which the individual takes her identity. Defences have a role in maintaining some degree of functioning of the person. That functioning may be dysfunctional. However, it is the best that person has managed to achieve given their particular set of experiencing and the conditions of worth that have influenced the development of their self-structure. They will still seek to defend it until such time as they feel ready to risk change. Often this is when the discomfort that comes from trying to maintain something outweighs the discomfort associated with the perceived risk of addressing it.

His mind also fleetingly went back to the last session when Mandy had said she felt alone when she was crying and feeling the loss of her mother. That phrase 'good to know I am not alone' suddenly had a deeper significance and he felt the urge to reflect it back to Mandy. He was also aware that he still didn't really know what she had meant by 'weird'. He was about to say something when Mandy continued.

'Yes, it's good to not feel alone.' It was said with a lot of feelings that were contrary to what the words implied. Mandy was back with feeling alone. She tightened her lips. 'I've got to get on with my life, accept it as it is, and make the best of things.'

'That was said with a lot of feeling: "I've got to get on with my life, accept it as it is, and make the best of things."' Martin spoke slowly and deliberately, allowing Mandy to really hear what she had just said.

She nodded. 'Yes, and that's just what I am doing. Yes, I can feel alone, and I don't like it, but it's the way things are at the moment. I've got my job, I have a nice home, good friends, and I'm discovering a new me as well. And who knows? Anyway, I do want to spend time reflecting on work and how I am doing. I don't want to get into anything heavy in this session. I'm sure that I could, I know that I have things from my past to sort out, but not now. I want to put my energy into establishing who I am, what I want and how I am going to get it.'

Martin went to say something, intending to empathise with what Mandy had just said, but she continued.

'I am not going to be busy all the time, I am going to learn to relax more and I am going to get out and about more with friends, get more of a social life. Work has taken over for too long. I want to live a little.'

Mandy's words came across very strongly to Martin. He responded, 'That sounds pretty affirming.'

'Yes, it is. I really have had enough of work taking over. I am determined to break up that old pattern. When I talk about it, like I am doing now, I actually feel quite a surge of energy. I've already started making changes to my routine and it feels good. It feels liberating and I want more of it. It really feels as though I am putting down some heavy weight, or rather, I have put it down, and now I have to avoid picking the damn thing up again.'

Martin nodded. 'Mhmm. Determined. Liberating. Want to avoid picking it up again.'

'And I'm *not* going to.' Mandy's voice had become very strong. 'Time to get a life outside of work. Not that I haven't had a life, but I really feel that it has taken over the last few years and I'm going to push it back. So I've started to plan how to change the times that I travel in to work, try to avoid traffic and be in less of a rush. I want to get home a little earlier some evenings by starting earlier, then I can do something with my time.'

'Do something with your time,' Martin couldn't help emphasising the 'do'.

Not exactly empathic, but given the issue that Mandy has been bringing to counselling, it is perhaps not unreasonable for Martin to emphasise the 'do'. Strictly speaking this could be regarded as being directive. However, it is keeping to the client's frame of reference, although in a sense expanding it to include the context of what has been discussed before.

'Yes, but not a busy doing. I might relax, I might go out, I might watch something on TV. But it's going to be something planned, or something that I feel I want to do. It's like giving myself permission, somehow.' Mandy stopped and thought about it for a moment. 'Yes, giving myself permission.'

'Permission to. . . ?' Martin replied.

'Permission to do what *I* want to do. I've run around too much for work. I am going to start to take care of myself more. I have begun to cut back on the processed foods and am making time to cook fresh vegetables. I am going to take care of my health and wellbeing. I owe it to myself. I feel that I deserve something better.' Mandy smiled, although she still looked very serious. 'Yes, it is time to change, and change I shall achieve. Carry on the way I have been and, well, at least my blood pressure is down a bit now. But I have got to reduce stress and pressure and that is what I am going to do.'

'So, you're going to look after yourself and it sounds like you really value your health and wellbeing.'

'I do. I've let it slip, and I've got to take more responsibility, make time for myself.'

'Put yourself, your needs, your health and wellbeing more centre stage.' Martin was aware of really trying to summarise the last two comments Mandy had made.

'Yes, and, you know, it is amazing. I mean, I came here, what, six or seven weeks ago, knowing things weren't right but not really with any idea about anything, as it turns out. And I have found myself weeping buckets, experiencing all kinds of feelings and memories and somehow, out of all of that, here I am contemplating ... no, not contemplating, actually making big changes to my routines. I can't really explain it, but that's what's happening.'

Martin smiled. It wasn't for him to start explaining theory.

Mandy has felt accepted. She has been allowed to express her innermost feelings on various experiences in her life. She has felt listened to and heard. Her pain has felt validated and respected. She has not been pushed or directed into any particular attitude or action. She has been allowed to experience herself, perhaps more fully than ever before.

As a result, she has released herself from attitudes and behaviours rooted in past conditioning. She has, in a sense, re-evaluated her sense of self and has realised that there is more to her, and to life, than what was previously present. The striving for greater control over her working life and life in general, of finding time to relax and to make her own choices has become attractive to her. She senses that it will give her satisfaction. It might be said that a new part or 'configuration within self' is emerging. This configuration has not been named but it seems to contain elements of taking care of her health and wellbeing, of seeking relaxation, of being less driven by unrealistic demands of herself. These activities and behaviours, when performed, bring a sense of satisfaction and a feel-good factor. She will therefore seek to continue with these behaviours in order to maintain these satisfying feelings.

We might view this in terms of Mandy's actualising tendency finding focus through this new configuration, extending her sense of self and enabling her to recreate significant elements within her structure of self.

Martin nodded and simply responded with, 'Changes, big changes. It has been quite a journey for you, but you are aware of profound shifts and changes within yourself. And it's hard to understand how it has happened, but you know that you are different.'

'Yes,' Mandy replied, while thinking how good it felt, and how much more energised she was feeling for talking about it. 'I feel much more energised than when I came in as well.' She smiled, and thinking about this her mind went back to what she had wanted to talk about. 'Which reminds me, I really did want to check out what I have been experiencing at work this week, so can we take some time for that? I realise that time is passing.'

'Sure.' Martin was aware that he was also feeling good about what Mandy had achieved and he wanted to voice this and communicate to her how he felt before she moved on. 'Before looking at what has been happening for you at work, I do want to say that I am pleased that you have a sense of having changed in a positive manner over the last few weeks. It makes me feel really pleased, really happy for you.' He was aware of a sense of excitement, 'And it feels kind of exciting somehow, a sort of new beginning. So I am interested to hear what you have done at the start of this new beginning.' He hadn't planned to say anything about a new beginning, it just seemed to flow from what he was saying.

'I suppose I hadn't really thought of it quite like that and yet that is what it is, a new beginning, a kind of fresh start. Yes, that really helps me to somehow get a clearer sense of me. I am seeking a fresh start. A new me and a fresh start. Yes.' Mandy smiled. 'Yes.' She was aware of looking a little bit into the distance, her thoughts had drifted off towards an unknown future. She was aware that she didn't really know what was going to happen in her life, and it felt OK. Something in her made her feel that perhaps it was scary and she should be anxious, but she didn't feel that way.

Martin was aware that Mandy seemed to have drifted off after that last 'yes'. He commented, 'You seem to have drifted off on to a train of thought somewhere.'

'Mhmm? Oh yes, sorry. Funny that. Just started thinking about the future and feeling I should be anxious, but I'm not. But I don't want to get into that just now.'

'Don't want to get into that now?'

'No.'

'OK. You were saying you wanted to focus on your experience since you've been back.' Martin was also conscious that time was passing, that it was the last session and he wondered what kind of ending Mandy would feel she needed. In a way he kind of felt that her summing up a few minutes ago of what she had achieved had been a kind of review that was part of the ending process. Ah well, he thought, I'm sure she knows what she needs to focus on, so I really should put my thoughts about endings aside.

While counselling is a process with various stages, not all clients experience or express a desire to spend time on endings. This may be because they are uncomfortable, or they could simply want to keep to some other more pressing focus. Mandy has revealed sensitivity to loss and so her ending with Martin could have a significant effect on her, given the role he has played in the changes she has made. However, as a person-centred counsellor Martin is unlikely to introduce the idea of some ritualistic ending process. He will honour the client's prioritising. He will seek to maintain his empathy for whatever she is experiencing and communicating to him.

Martin is aware that Mandy appreciates what the counselling has given her. However, he is likely to be mindful of her experiences of loss and therefore out of respect for her as a person is likely to convey his feelings towards the end of the session, but in a way that will be supportive to the client and not blow the ending out of all proportion. He will trust implicitly her inner wisdom and the flow of her actualising tendency into the areas of her self that are growing and developing, although he will be aware too that those aspects of her nature that she is seeking to leave behind may strike back at some point (Mearns, 1992) and may raise this concern out of his compassion and caring for her future wellbeing.

'It's not that I have a lot to say, but I feel good about the changes I have been making and want to share them. It's nice to have something positive to talk about.'

'Nice to have something to feel positive about to bring here and talk about.'

'Yes, it's a good feeling.' Mandy took a moment to reflect back to Monday. 'Well, I went back Monday and I was feeling a bit anxious, you know, not sure what people might think with me being away for a few weeks, and not sure how I would react. I felt stronger inside and determined not to slide back into my old pattern. My boss was really understanding and said he didn't want me to rush into too much, but to build up gradually. So that was encouraging.'

'Mhmm. Bit anxious but feeling stronger and encouraged by your boss's reaction,' Martin reflected back.

Mandy nodded. 'So I told him that I planned to vary my working times to reduce traffic delays, and my idea of bringing my team together more often and spending less time myself driving from place to place. I argued that it would be good for my team members to have more contact with each other, kind of bond them a bit more. I was really surprised when he suggested that maybe we needed an away-day to take time out to reflect on our teams' values and goals, and to help them contribute their ideas as well.'

Martin had noted that Mandy's voice seemed to be conveying surprise, and he reflected this back to her. 'I sense that you sound surprised by this.'

'I was. It seems, though, that there have been some discussions at higher management level. Lots of concerns about the numbers of people who do not stay long with the company. It seems that my absence was another statistic which contributed to this process. Seems that there is a bit of a culture change happening. So that is really, really encouraging.'

'Yes, I can hear that note of enthusiasm in your voice.'

'Well, I do feel enthusiastic, but I am also a little cautious as well. I've been in the company a few years now and there is a cynical part of me that wonders just how long this will last. But I want to put that aside and give it a chance. So I have been giving thought the last two days to ways of bringing my team together, and I am excited by this. In fact, I have decided to bring in an outside facilitator for part of the day which I hope will be fun. I don't want it all to be too serious. I like the people in my team, they are good at what they do. Of course, they're all different, but, yeah, it feels like a new energy, new possibilities. Feels like there's going to be some creative space.' Mandy had been so surprised when she had got back and to hear what her boss was saying. She felt swept up by it and really wanted to get into it. She'd spent both evenings this week thinking about it at home as well.

'Creative space, that sounds quite a contrast to the treadmill that you had been on, and the busy-ness that you want to get away from.'

'Yes, I'm really up for it. Been spending my evenings planning for it and thinking about possible developments in the team.'

Both evenings, Martin thought, and he wondered where Mandy's plan to not take work home had gone. Yet he was also aware of her energy and enthusiasm and wanted to be sure of honouring this as it was this aspect that she was communicating and therefore wanting him to hear.

'Both evenings?' he asked, aware that it was a bit of a loaded question, but he wanted to hold Mandy on this to give her an opportunity to explore how she felt about this.

'Ye-es. Why?' Mandy was initially puzzled and then it dawned on her. 'Oh, you think I'm "busying" again?'

Martin did wonder about this, although he had noted to himself that it had felt different. He sought to reflect in his response exactly how he was feeling, it was important to be open and honest. He was expecting this of Mandy.

The honesty and transparency of the counsellor in these situations is of vital therapeutic importance. Whether it is the start of a therapeutic relationship, or it is drawing near to a close, the core conditions are important and the counsellor must seek to offer them to the best of his ability.

'I have to say I wonder, Mandy, but I also want to honour your enthusiasm, which doesn't sound like the driven need to be busy you spoke about in earlier sessions. I guess I'm checking it out, partly for me, no, maybe mainly for me, but partly for you. I'm sitting here aware that this is our last session and, well, I want to feel that you will go away from here giving yourself every opportunity to create the lifestyle, work pattern, etc., that you really want for yourself.' He felt a warmth for Mandy and wanted to convey this. He was also aware that he had kind of drifted into a bit of a monologue. But he was aware of feeling that he wanted to try and be sure Mandy had all the angles covered, as it were. And he also knew that wasn't possible, and that he really should trust her to make her own choices, choices that would be right for her.

'I hear what you say, and I did question myself at one point on the Monday evening. I was scribbling down ideas at the kitchen table, and I remember looking up at the clock and thinking, "Ten o'clock, where's the evening gone?" And then almost immediately the thought cut in "Where's *my* evening gone?" I did stop and think about it, did a kind of reality check on myself. Was I working away because of a drive to be busy, did I feel pushed into it by my boss and felt unable to say no, or did it feel like a choice, a free choice, of my own? I came to the conclusion that it was my choice and that it felt good. However, it was at that point as well that I decided to stop for the evening. And I felt good about it. The next evening I didn't work on it so late, and I took time out to watch the first of a new crime series on TV. I also gave myself time both evenings to prepare and cook a meal. So I *am* looking after myself.' Mandy felt a sense of having to justify herself sweep through her, and she really didn't like it. Felt like she was having to explain herself. She was aware she had frowned slightly and tightened her lips.

Martin noticed her changed facial expression. He was sitting feeling as if he was being reported to, and it didn't feel right for him either. 'Feels like you are reporting back to me on your homework. I hadn't meant for that to happen, at least, I wasn't consciously asking for that.'

'Yes, it does, and I seem to have been happy to do it as well!' Mandy shook her head. 'And I felt like I was justifying myself.' She was still shaking her head. She stopped and thought for a moment.

'Justifying yourself?' Martin had responded.

'Yes, still having to justify myself, get brownie points, show that I'm good enough. I walked into that, didn't I.' Mandy was smiling again. 'I really walked into that. I feel comfortable about.... I'm doing it again. I don't have to justify myself to you. I damn well know it felt good, that I *was* taking care of myself.' Mandy had raised her voice. She was feeling quite angry, or was it anger? Was she simply feeling assertive? It had suddenly risen up inside her. She thought about it. 'Yes, angry, but in an assertive kind of way.'

'Really makes you feel quite angry having to justify yourself to me, and you really want to assert yourself, that you can trust your own judgement on this. You knew it felt good and you knew you were taking care of yourself.' Martin could sense the anger and the link to justification, though part of him was wondering whether Mandy was justifying herself to him or to herself. But it did not seem pressing and . . . Mandy was speaking again.

'I don't need to justify it, I know what I was feeling.' She noticed Martin was smiling now. 'What the hell are you smiling at?'

Martin broke out into a broad grin. 'I'm sorry, well, I'm not really, but I want to say how much I really value and appreciate hearing you tell me that you don't have to justify it, that you know what you were feeling, and that's good enough. It feels good to hear you say that. Yeah, you know what you felt, what you were experiencing, and you knew you were making a choice, or choices, satisfying to you.' Martin genuinely felt that something had moved on for Mandy. She was claiming, owning, a strong belief in herself, and in her ability to evaluate her own motivations. He felt somehow more comfortable, as if some inner tension that he had been carrying had released itself.

Mandy smiled too. Yes, I do feel that I have moved on. And it does feel positive. I know it's early days, but I feel different and ready to embrace new possibilities.' She glanced at the clock and noticed that there were fewer than ten minutes left.

Mandy's ability to evaluate her experience for herself has been validated. She has made a powerful affirmation here. Her locus of evaluation has been internalised on this issue, and she is quite adamant about this and is quite vocal in defending it.

While some counsellors might question whether she is being defensive, and maybe isn't feeling so convinced in herself as she makes out, the person-centred counsellor is much more likely to trust the client and enable her to affirm her evaluation. The person-centred counsellor is only likely to question it if he is experiencing a powerful internal reaction himself that he senses to be relevant to the relationship, and which he feels needs to be congruently voiced.

Martin noticed her glance. 'Yes, just a few more minutes. I also sense a moving on, and I want to acknowledge and celebrate it.' Martin paused, unsure what to say next and being aware that he wanted to let Mandy decide how to use the last few minutes of time they had together within the therapeutic relationship. 'And I wonder how you want to use the last few minutes?'

Mandy stopped and thought. It had been quite a few weeks. She really did feel different and was very grateful. 'I want to say thanks for giving me your time and the opportunity to go through what has happened for me these last few weeks. You have been a steadying influence somehow, sort of reliable, but more than that. I felt that you somehow trusted me, trusted..., I don't know, but there was a kind of calmness. I wasn't hurried, I felt accepted. Yes, I felt accepted, even just now when I got angry, somehow it was OK. You didn't get defensive. In fact, you just smiled. But it was a warm smile, a kind of accepting smile.' Mandy stopped for a moment and thought. Yes, it was being accepted, feeling accepted for who she was. 'It all felt reassuring even though I was experiencing so much hurt at times. And I felt really good being angry just now as well. I couldn't have done that seven weeks ago, at least, not without feeling awful about it afterwards.'

The session has very definitely moved into an ending with a period of reflection on what the therapeutic journey has meant for Mandy and Martin. This is quite an important step. It generates a kind of mutuality in the relationship. It enables the client to experience the therapeutic relationship very much on an adult-to-adult basis, as two people who have shared a set of experiences together. During the counselling, clients can experience a degree of dependence on the counsellor. In this ending process the client is affirming her identity and her independence.

It can also stand out in stark relief and given the setting. Such a 'feeling-centred' 'conversation' is far less likely between a patient and another healthcare professional.

The interaction in the next few minutes does become more conversational, again offering a moving-on experience for client and counsellor. The counselling connection has ended. Two people are together ending (both client *and* counsellor are experiencing an ending process) a set of shared experiencing. It will have been helpful for the client to affirm for herself the positive changes she has made and which she will be carrying into her life over the coming weeks and beyond.

Martin appreciated what Mandy had said and was pleased that she had experienced these qualities. He particularly appreciated the fact that she felt accepted. He wanted to reinforce this. 'Well, I feel grateful for what you have told me. I certainly sought to accept you, and I wanted to accept you. I wanted to be with you as a companion on this, what shall I call it, therapeutic journey? It seems to me that a number of difficult areas in your experiencing got uncovered, and yet you bravely, and I want to say courageously, persevered.'

'Stubborn,' Mandy replied with a smile.

'You may say stubborn, OK, but I think it takes a lot of courage to face up to and embrace painful feelings. I know sometimes it feels as though we don't have much choice in the matter, but you kept coming back for more. And I respect that.' Martin was aware of feeling a bit of a lump in his throat as he said that. He was speaking from the heart and he knew it. 'Yeah, I want to respect your courage and I want to wish you the very best for the future.'

Mandy could feel herself getting a little tearful. Hearing Martin talk about his respect for her courage was something no one had ever said to her before. It felt strange, yet somehow there seemed to be a warm glow within the strangeness. Somewhere, deep inside, she sensed that there was courage. It seemed like a small spark but maybe her task was to fan that spark into a flame.

'Thank you for that.' Mandy suddenly felt a sense of the loneliness of walking out of the door. Her mind went back to the conversation they had had when she had raised the issue of further counselling beyond six sessions. 'And if I want more counselling at some point?'

'Refer yourself back to Dr Hill. Discuss the options with her.'

'And if I wanted something over a longer period of time?'

'Dr Hill will discuss where you could be referred, and what options there are either within the NHS or privately. If you decide you want private counselling she will give you a list of local counsellors and details of national registers of counsellors.' Martin was keeping it general. He knew it was not for him to promote his own private practice. If Mandy wished to approach him about that then they would need to discuss it at the time.

'And if I wanted a longer period of counselling with you? I mean, you appreciate where I am coming from and I wouldn't really want to start again with someone else.'

'I do appreciate that and I hear what you say. But you would need to go back to Dr Hill and discuss what you feel you need. She will then pass on details of counsellors, including mine, and you can then make your own decision if that is what you feel you want to do at some point.'

'OK. I'm not thinking of straight away. I want to see how things work out. But it would be good to know what the procedure is.'

'It's important that you are given a range of options if you want further counselling, particularly if you want to go outside the NHS. It would be unethical for me to encourage you to see me specifically, yeah?'

'I do understand.'

It is important that counsellors do not and are not seen to promote their own private practice. Referring the matter back to the GP, and the GP having a range of options for the client who wants longer-term, private counselling, is ethically sound.

'Oh, I need to give you this feedback sheet. If you'd like to complete it and return it to the surgery sometime, it would be helpful. It's confidential, no names mentioned, but an opportunity for you to feed back to the surgery your feelings about the counselling, whether or not it was helpful, that kind of thing.'

'Sure.' Mandy took a deep breath, and held out her hand. 'Well, thanks for everything. More than anything, thanks for *listening*.'

'It's what we counsellors do best. It's been good knowing you and working with you. Take care of yourself and every good wish for your future.'

'Thanks.' Mandy turned and exited through the counselling room door. She felt a range of feelings: a sadness at ending, yet a determination to make the counselling count for something in her life. She thought she might like more counselling but not just yet. She was much more aware of herself, and knew that she had to make her own way forward. But it had been helpful. She knew she felt different about herself, and felt more able to be herself. It had been a liberating experience and now she had to move on. She glanced at her watch. She was meeting a friend in half an hour, time to get over to the car park on the other side of town and to meet her outside her office. She felt a mixture of thoughtfulness and yet somewhat carefree as well as she got into her car and fired the engine into life. Yes, she thought, it's my life and I *am* going to live it *my* way.

Client case notes

Client recognises her difficulty in accepting positive feedback from others about herself. Affirms that she wants to get on with her life and that she feels she is giving herself permission to do what she wants to do. Reflected on her few days at work, feels she is making progress at making the changes she wants. Client again asked about longer-term private counselling and has been advised to discuss with her GP. Client has not been given private contact details of the counsellor.

Points for discussion/action

- Mandy says at one point that 'it's good to feel not alone' and this is not reflected back by Martin. Why do you think this might be? Was it a mistake? How else might Martin have responded?
- Reflect on the significance and impact of Martin's congruent expression within this session.
- Is the listening ability of a counsellor the most important factor?
- What issues do you think Martin might now take to supervision from this final session?
- Make your own notes for this session.
- Critically evaluate the ending process within the context of person-centred working.

In counselling there are often key moments that provide opportunity for a client to, for instance, engage with an aspect of herself that is important, see something from a fresh perspective, or maybe affirm an aspect of herself that is emerging into being. Good counselling involves the ability to be attentive to these key moments. They are rather like 'big points' that the really good tennis players tend to win, and the not-so-good players are inconsistent on. The really effective counsellor will be particularly 'tuned in' when these moments arise.

You cannot prepare for them as they can arise at any time. But if you are maintaining empathy for your client, a sensitivity towards your own inner experiencing that is then offered congruently, and are holding a warm and accepting attitude of unconditional positive regard for the client as a person, then you are more likely to recognise them and respond in a manner that is helpful to the client.

- Reflect on the whole counselling process. Pick out three significant moments that were of particular therapeutic value and discuss why you have chosen them.

Reflection

Martin liked to take time to reflect on the process and on his feelings and thoughts after ending with a client. It was frequently such a poignant time. His senses were often heightened and it was an opportunity to gain insight into his own process and the nature of the therapeutic relationship while it was very much present for him.

He felt that he had really engaged with Mandy. He felt good about that. It was a fulfilling and satisfying experience to end a series of counselling sessions feeling that therapeutic alliance had been established. The cost of this, as he knew, was that it could leave him feeling a little sad. He had been a companion with Mandy on a very emotional journey, and it had affected him. He had been deeply touched by the emotions she had brought into the relationship.

He felt that she had moved on significantly. He now felt that her confidence was genuine. He was aware, however, that powerful feelings remained and that they would still affect Mandy at times. Do we ever truly leave these kinds of feeling behind somehow, or do we take them with us, he pondered? He felt Mandy was stronger and more resilient. Yet he was also aware that she was undertaking the changing of patterns of behaviour that had become established early in life.

He was impressed by the wide range of issues that had come to light during the sessions. As he reflected back, particular episodes came to mind: the dissociation to her four-year-old self; her sadness and loneliness following the death of her mother, and her desperate wanting to thank her mother; her struggle to free herself from her busy-ness; her determination to assert herself as a woman with her own power; her practical session planning the changes she would make at work.

Martin smiled to himself as he thought about how unstructured the sessions had been, how much he had sought to allow Mandy the space to direct her therapy. She had got to where she needed to be in those sessions. He believed strongly that he could trust his clients to use the sessions, particularly when they were clear as to the time they had. Mandy had worked, really worked, and had kept coming back for more when she might have decided it was too painful.

His sense was that clients did best when they were in a place in themselves that left them ready to address issues, even though to begin with they may not be fully aware of exactly what needed to be addressed. People couldn't really be prescribed counselling, like other treatments, unless they were motivated to attend. Yet he could remember instances where clients had come not knowing much about why they had been referred and had ended up benefiting greatly. So often it came back down to people feeling listened to. This came over strongly on his feedback forms. Being listened to and being given time. He smiled. So much emphasis on 'talking therapies', but surely the value is as much, if not more, on the 'listening' aspect of the therapy and on the client feeling heard.

So, Mandy had returned to work and was putting her plans into action. He hoped they would be sustainable. She was obviously committed to her work but was also now becoming increasingly committed to seeking out experiences that brought her a sense of fulfilment. What was it she had said? Something about wanting 'time for myself'. He hoped she would find it. What he had no doubt about was that within her nature Mandy had that 'actualising tendency' that Rogers wrote of (Rogers, 1961) and that whatever path she took it would be urging her to grow and to develop as a person in her own right. Martin wasn't sure that we ever reached that, but that life was about the journey, the striving to become the person that we have the potential for being.

He had written his notes and he closed the file, preparing to take it back to the locked cabinet. He thought for a moment about the awesome power of offering a therapeutic climate, and of the impact that congruence, empathy and unconditional positive regard could have on people who were in a state of incongruence or anxiety. In one sense it seemed so simple, yet he knew that the discipline of achieving these attitudinal qualities within the session was highly demanding, and that being a person-centred counsellor was a commitment to life-long learning (Thorne, 2002b) in order to ensure that he could offer his clients the quality of presence that presented the opportunity for constructive personality change.

Conclusion

It is my hope that this book has raised a number of issues regarding working in a time limited context from the perspective of the PCA.

There is a growing tendency for counsellors working as time limited therapists to have to demonstrate that they have clear and specific goals for their clients for each session, and that they can therefore comment on each session as to how or whether these goals were achieved. This approach, with the counsellor knowing in advance precisely what the client's needs are in a particular session, is completely contrary to a person-centred way of working.

The person-centred counsellor enters into a therapeutic relationship with a client with the intention of being attentive to whatever the client brings to the session and to the relationship. There is no goal for a particular session, or indeed for a series of sessions, other than that which the client brings. This is fundamental. It lies at the heart of the PCA, the trust that the client knows what they need to address, what is most urgent and pressing for them, given the context of a limited time frame to work in.

Added to this is the fact that people change during the therapeutic process and factors can arise that were previously not known by the client or linked by them to the difficulty that she is seeking to resolve. One cannot know, at the outset, all the factors that are linked to the presenting issue. The client may not appreciate at the outset the depth of feeling that she may associate with particular experiences that has relevance to the difficulty that has caused her to seek, or be referred, to counselling.

What is being sought within person-centred counselling is a quality of relationship. The client is being allowed space, albeit time limited, in which aspects of herself – feelings, thoughts, behaviours – can arise and be made visible. The client may then communicate these to the counsellor, or she may not. That is the client's choice. For sensitive matters to be communicated the client will need to feel she can trust the counsellor, and the build up of this trust can take time. Within time limited working it is quite possible that the client will not experience that depth of trust in the therapeutic relationship needed to disclose something. It will depend on the individual, the experiences that she has faced and quite possibly on the degree of emotional pain or mental anguish that she is carrying. There are clients who will need time to trust their counsellor (particularly where trust is a component of the underlying issue) and others who are simply at bursting point and just have to talk and have their story heard by someone, anyone, who appears to be offering them time and attention within an atmosphere of non-judgemental, warm acceptance.

To create the necessary therapeutic environment for the client to trust the counsellor with their inner world requires the client to be offered a therapeutic and relational environment in which the client experiences a certain freedom to be herself, to make discoveries, to experiment with new ways of being or to engage with a fresh perspective on how she currently experiences herself and her inner world. The goal, if there is a goal in person-centred counselling, is simply the creation of this facilitative climate. There is not, however, a goal held by the person-centred counsellor to make a particular something happen within that climate of therapeutic relationship.

The factor of freedom is an important one. The recognition that the client has within herself a tendency towards actualisation which, given a warm and accepting environment, can be trusted to direct the client towards an increasingly realistic perspective on herself and her situation is a crucial feature of person-centred theory. Rogers makes it clear that in his view 'individuals have within themselves vast resources for self-understanding and for altering their self-concepts, basic attitudes and self-directed behaviour; these resources can be tapped if a definable climate of facilitative psychological attitudes can be provided' (Rogers, 1980, p.115). The person-centred counsellor trusts the client's own process, recognising that this may lead to the resolution of the difficulty through the therapeutic encounter, and/or it may leave the client deciding to make changes in her life in order to generate a greater sense of satisfaction and fulfilment which then contributes to the resolution of what has become a problem for her. Of course, it may not be a matter of change as the solution. For the client, the sense of achievement may come through reaching a place of genuine and informed acceptance of a situation, or of aspects of herself that she was previously fighting which left her in a place of inner tension and conflict.

Symptoms only tell us so much. In some counselling contexts where there is a time limited focus, the NHS, EAPs and other workplace schemes, for instance, there can be a strong element of the person being referred in order to resolve not only a specifically diagnosed problem, but also in a particular way. Perhaps a stressed client is referred in order to manage her stress more effectively, or a sacked client in order to learn to accept what has happened; a depressed client might be referred with the goal that she might be made to feel happier about her life, or the anxious person to learn to be more at ease with life. These are reasonable goals in one sense. However, they may not necessarily be reasonable to the client. Psychological health is surely more than the eradication of symptoms. It is rather about understanding the context and enabling the client to be how she herself wishes to be, to express what feelings she may have or to take action that for whatever reason she had held back from because of her inner state of confusion and incongruence.

The stressed client mentioned above may well want to feel less stress, but the problem might not be so much their inability to manage or handle it, but rather it is a problem stemming from the organisation they work from, which places unrealistic demands and has unrealistic expectations of staff. So, healthy counselling that is open to the client's own needs and process could well mean that rather than the client seeking to manage stress, they might become more aware of their feelings about how they have been treated and either seek to change the organisation or seek alternative employment, or initiate a complaint against the company.

For the anxious client, there may be a goal of reducing the anxiety. The tranquillisers have not worked, or perhaps they left the client so tranquillised that she found this unacceptable. Perhaps, however, the client is a member of a marginalised group within society and feels threatened as a result. Maybe this client is also very aware of the ecological disaster that the world seems to be heading towards and feels it deeply. For her there is a deep fear of the future. Some might consider this anxiety to be unrealistic, but is it? Is it a condition to be treated, or is it an experience that is appropriate to circumstances? Within the person-centred counselling sessions the client becomes more in touch with these feelings and decides that rather than try to suppress them, a more satisfying response would be to act on them, to use the anxious energy in some constructive manner. Managing them or subduing them through medication become potential constraints. Perhaps the client chooses to become politically active, finding a fulfilment in this that is truly a life-changing experience.

The depressed client in a GP surgery may be referred by the GP who wants her to become more accepting of something in her life and to become more motivated to take an interest in her family. However, the client's depression may actually be the result of feelings of being totally powerless within the family structure. The client may have had similar experiences in childhood and has chosen a relationship for herself that maintains that state of powerlessness. However, she has matured and is aware that this choice was rooted in conditioning, and is realising that there is more to her and to life, and is depressed because she feels unable to do anything about it. As the person-centred counselling proceeds, the client revisits those early life experiences and recognises the pattern that she has been living out. She realises that she has 'forgotten' much of what she had experienced. At first, as it all rises into awareness, the depression deepens. Medically, it would seem the depression is not being cured, the counselling isn't working, something else must be done. However, the reality is that the client is gaining an increasingly authentic view of her past and experiencing a natural and normal reaction.

Seeing it from the angle of an adult, she is angry and feels strong motivation to change. Her experience of unconditional positive regard from the counsellor offers her the therapeutic climate to grow in new ways. She makes her own connections and perhaps the part, or configuration within self, that is rooted in an 'I must satisfy my need to feel powerless because that is normal' experience begins to weaken. An 'I am powerful' part begins to emerge and it feels increasingly satisfying. It could be the first time this experience has been allowed to be present, previously it has been defended against to maintain the sense of powerlessness. The client may be left feeling appropriately angry towards what she experienced in the past, and in the present. She may no longer wish to remain in a relationship which was based on a need to satisfy that aspect of her sense of self that needed to feel powerless.

By not having an agenda or goal to lift the client's mood by seeking only behavioural and cognitive changes, but rather being open to the client's own experiencing and connections, an opportunity has been created for this client to explore and establish a new way of being that has been, if you like, organically grown within a therapeutically and psychologically healthy climate of relationship. The counsellor has not sought to 'do' anything or to 'treat' specific symptoms, but the outcome is a person who has cleared away limiting psychological patterns from her past and who is learning to embrace a new way of being. It is then for the client to decide how she will be within her circumstances and what changes she may, or may not, choose to make. Whatever she decides, it will have its roots in a much more healthy and authentic/congruent state.

These examples, I believe, indicate how we need to look beyond symptoms and to offer clients space to develop in the freeing atmosphere of a person-centred relationship. The counsellor, working in a time limited way, will need to be aware that the process that will bring clients to what is a satisfying outcome for them cannot be artificially compressed into a 'one-size-fits-all' service. We can also not foretell what may arise within the counselling sessions, however in-depth (and therefore frequently invasive) an assessment process might be. Yet the reality of time limited working remains and it is my experience that clients do adapt to this time frame and work within it to the depth that they feel able to manage. Occasionally, a client's deep trauma and distress may emerge and clearly further therapeutic involvement is required, and flexibility is required to offer more sessions to either deal with what has emerged, or to prepare the client for a referral on for a more lengthy process.

In the counselling sessions in this book it is clear that there are potentially difficult underlying issues that have not been addressed fully: the separation and being fostered by relatives as a child; the patterns and meanings established in Mandy's mind; and emotions in response to her mother's emphasis on work. There is also the question of whether Mandy's 'please don't make me' response is simply her response to being taken from her mother, or whether, as Martin had initially assumed and anticipated, there might have been a childhood sexual abuse issue present (often referred to as CSA, a sanitising acronym that causes us to avoid saying it as it is). This, however, did not emerge. This does not mean that it did not happen, we simply do not know. But if it did occur, and the memories are deeply forgotten, then I would take the view that the time was not right. Martin and Mandy worked with what was brought into the presence of the relationship and their individual awarenesses. For Martin to have pursued his wonder and to have pushed Mandy on this would have brought it to the surface at a time that was out of step with Mandy's own psychological and emotional process. The person-centred counsellor trusts that the client's essential personhood, the structure of self that has been developed through a lifetime of experience, will know what it needs to do in order to be psychologically effective. When the structure of self is under strain, when it can no longer hold back memories, when the little voice that is calling for help is finally heard, *then* the time is right for it to begin to emerge into the client's awareness. It is then the time to deal with it.

For Mandy, within the time frame she has been given for counselling, she has perhaps gone as far as she feels able to go, or maybe able to risk going. She has done enough to enable her to release feelings and to recognise her need for change. She has taken action and is working at establishing a new work pattern, and a social life, to satisfy the person she has become through the counselling process. She may have gone back to work sooner in order to fit in with having that final session after her return, and this may have been premature. Yet it may have been right for her at that time. We cannot be sure. Only time will tell.

Perhaps Mandy may never need to seek counselling again. The work she has done may have been enough to enable her to establish a new attitude and work pattern, and so enable her to enter into a new cycle within her life leading to … well, we can only guess. Maybe less work and more play may lead to romance. Or travel. Or new experiences that lead to new opportunities and further changes.

Then again, Mandy may find that she cannot sustain her change of attitude, and her work once again gets on top of her. She may then return for further counselling and this may involve her working more deeply, or it could be that she needs to take time to explore her options and make other changes: of job or career.

What would have been different had Mandy been offered open-ended counselling, or an agreed larger number of sessions? Would the process have been different? Would the outcome have been different? This is speculative. We can never be sure how a client will react to the time frame offered to them. An open-ended counselling contract may have meant that Mandy would relax and feel less pressured (if in fact she did) to get on with what she felt she needed to do. This may have meant more time for reflection and exploration within sessions, but equally the reduced sense of intensity brought on by knowing that time was not limited might have some other effect on Mandy's motivation to work on herself.

The factor of time being limited may have left her feeling that she had to seek a successful outcome (from her frame of reference) in order to generate a sense of satisfaction and achievement, which are experiences that would probably be important to her. Certainly, it is likely that she would not have gone back to work so soon had there been more sessions available. But whether her process of actualising would have left her dwelling further and more deeply on some of the issues that arose, we can only guess.

Personally, I think that time limited counselling does generate the possibility of an enhanced sense of focus for the client (and for the therapist). The question remains, however, whether the results of the counselling will be sustainable over time. Does the length of time for counselling correlate with what the client perceives as a successful outcome? It seems likely that it is perhaps quality rather than quantity of counselling that is more crucial, but the length of time has to be a significant factor too. There are many variables.

There will also be those for whom the thought of months if not years of therapy is the last thing they wish to contemplate. For them, the choice of being able to move in and out of therapy for brief periods as the need arises is much more acceptable. They may regard therapy as being rather like taking a car in for a service, an opportunity to focus on resolving anything particular that is problematic or threatening to be so, and to generally check that all is well.

Yet it is not only the client who is likely to be affected by the factor of limited time. What of the counsellor? Martin is aware that he finds it hard to work with, and this theme arises in his supervision. He is likely therefore to be carrying extra tension, but what is important is that he is aware of it. Does it affect how he works with Mandy? It is bound to, particularly where issues arise in the sessions that he feels might usefully be explored given more time. He does feel that the process is cut short, or rather accelerated towards the end. Yet he must also take care that his own anxiety does not cause him to try to hurry the client along. Mandy has to be allowed to journey at her own pace. Some clients will adapt to time limitation, sharpen up and in a sense 'get on with it'. Others will not do this, the limited time not being a factor for them, they will simply journey at their own pace through the time period offered. This could leave the counsellor frustrated if he feels that opportunity is being lost. But this is coming from his frame of reference and is his supervision if not therapy issue.

The person-centred therapist trusts his clients to know what they need to focus on, what is most pressing for them, what needs addressing within their inner world of experiencing. Insight and movement can come at any time within those six sessions (or between them of course). The challenge for the person-centred counsellor is to stay with the client, with their process, communicating as accurately as they can their empathic understanding of what the client is describing and bringing into the therapeutic relationship.

Final thoughts

Counselling is not a cure-all for life. It can never be that. It is an opportunity for people to explore, make sense of themselves and their experiences, and make decisions based on their developing sense of self. From a person-centred perspective it offers the opportunity for a person to feel heard and understood, to feel listened to, to experience being with someone who is striving to be congruent and authentic and to risk greater authenticity themselves, and to engage in a relationship with another person who offers them unconditional positive regard, warmth and prizing.

Time limited counselling provides people with a boundaried period in which to experience this climate of relationship. The client (and the counsellor) will be affected by the experience. Incongruencies within the client are likely to become more acutely experienced and demand attention. Problems may be resolved, some may become recognised as insoluble in such a short time frame. Either way, clients should be left with a clearer sense of self and a greater capacity to make authentic and satisfying choices in their lives.

References

Asay TP and Lambert MJ (1999) The empirical case for common factors in therapy. In: MA Hubble, BL Duncan and SD Miller (eds) *The Heart and Soul of Therapy*. American Psychological Association Press, Washington, DC.

British Association for Counselling and Psychotherapy (2000) *Information Sheet: Record Keeping and the Data Protection Act*. BACP, Rugby.

British Association for the Person Centred Approach (2000) *Client-centred Psychotherapy in the UK – the future*. Briefing paper. BAPCA, London.

Bentall RP (1990) The syndromes and symptoms of psychosis. In: RR Bentall (ed.) *Reconstructing Schizophrenia*. Routledge, London.

Bozarth J (1998) *Person-centered Therapy: a revolutionary paradigm*. PCCS Books, Ross-on-Wye.

Bozarth J (2002) Empirically supported treatments: epitome of the specificity myth. In: JC Watson, RN Goldman and MS Warner (eds) *Client-centred and Experiential Psychotherapy in the 21st Century: advances in theory research and practice*. PCCS Books, Ross-on-Wye, pp.168–81.

Bozarth J, Zimring FM, Tausch R (2002) Client-centred therapy: evolution of a revolution. In: D Caio and J Seeman (eds) *Handbook of Research and Practice in Humanistic Psychotherapies*. APA, Washington, DC.

Bryant-Jefferies R (1999) Sensory challenges to the primary health care client. *Counselling in Practice*, 3(1). Counselling in Primary Care Trust, Staines.

Casemore R (2000) Counselling challenge: time limits. *Counselling* 11(9): 543.

Casemore R (2002) It may be therapeutic but is it really counselling? *Healthcare Counselling and Psychotherapy Journal* 2(1): 6–8.

Curtis Jenkins G (2002) Good money after bad? The justification for the expansion of counselling services in primary health care. In: C Feltham (ed.) *What's the Good of Counselling & Psychotherapy?* Sage, London.

Hallam RS (1983) Agoraphobia: deconstructing a clinical syndrome. *Bulletin of the British Psychological Society* 36: 337–40.

Hallam RS (1989) Classification and research into panic. In: R Baker and M McFadyen (eds) *Panic Disorder*. Wiley, Chichester.

Hallet R (1990) *Melancholia and depression. A brief history and analysis of contemporary confusions*. Unpublished Masters thesis, University of East London.

Jenkins P (2002a) Whatever you say is confidential but ... *Counselling and Psychotherapy Journal* 13(2): 10–13.

Jenkins P (2002b) Shifting sands? Consent, confidentiality and date protection in the NHS. *Healthcare Counselling and Psychotherapy Journal* 2(2): 2–5.

King M, Sibbald B, Ward E, Bower P, Lloyd M, Gabbay M and Byford S (2000) Randomised control trial of non-directive counselling, cognitive behavioural therapy and usual general practitioner care in the management of depression as well as mixed anxiety and depression in primary care. *Health Technology Assessment* 4(19). Also published in the *British Medical Journal* 321: 1383–8.

Kutchins H and Kirk S (1997) *Making us Crazy: DSM: the psychiatric bible and the creation of mental disorders.* The Free Press/Simon Schuster, New York.

Mearns D (1992) On the self concept fighting back. In: W Dryden (ed.) *Hard Earned Lessons from Counselling in Action.* Sage, London.

Mearns D (2002) Response from the Lanarkshire Counselling Service. Letter published in *Healthcare Counselling and Psychotherapy Journal* 2(1): 2. BACP, Rugby.

Mearns D and Thorne B (1988) *Person Centred Counselling in Action.* Sage, London.

Mearns D and Thorne B (1999) *Person Centred Counselling in Action* (2e). Sage, London.

Mearns D and Thorne B (2000) *Person-centred Therapy Today: new frontiers in theory and practice.* Sage, London.

Merry T (2002) *Learning and Being in Person-centred Counselling* (2e). PCCS Books, Ross-on-Wye.

Miller SD, Duncan BL and Johnson LD (2001) Do patients want ineffective therapy? The undiscover'd country. *Counselling Practice* 5(2). Counselling in Primary Care Trust, Staines.

Palmer I and Mander G. *Time-limited to open-ended counselling – how to handle the transition.* BACP (British Association for Counselling and Psychotherapy). Information Sheet P3.

Richardson A (2001) Getting set for regulation. *Healthcare Counselling and Psychotherapy Journal* 1(2): 5–7.

Rogers CR (1951) *Client Centred Therapy.* Constable, London.

Rogers CR (1957) The necessary and sufficient conditions of therapeutic personality change. *Journal of Consulting Psychology* 21: 95–103.

Rogers CR (1961) *On Becoming a Person.* Constable, London.

Rogers CR (1980) *A Way of Being.* Houghton Mifflin, Boston, MA.

Rowland N, Mellor Clarke J, Bower P, Heywood P, Young P and Godfrey C (2000) Counselling for depression in primary care (protocol for a Cochrane review). *The Cochrane Library* 3. Update Software, Oxford.

Slade PD and Cooper R (1979) Some difficulties with the term 'schizophrenia': an alternative model. *British Journal of Social and Clinical Psychology* 18: 309–17.

Thorne B (2002a) Regulation – a treacherous path? *Counselling and Psychotherapy Journal* 13(2): 4–5. BACP, Rugby.

Thorne B (2002b) *The Mystical Power of the Person Centred Approach: hope beyond despair.* Whurr, London.

Warner MS (1991) Fragile process. In: L Fusek (ed.) *New Directions in Client-centered Therapy: practise with difficult client populations* (Monograph Series 1). Chicago Counselling and Psychotherapy Center, Chicago, IL, pp. 41–58.

Warner MS (1998) A client-centered approach to therapeutic work with dissociated and fragile process. In: L Greenberg, J Watson and G Lietaer (eds) *Handbook of Experiential Psychology*. Guildford Press, New York.

Warner MS (2000) Person-centred therapy at the difficult edge: a developmentally-based model of fragile and dissociated process. In: D Mearns and B Thorne (eds) *Person-centred Therapy Today: new frontiers in theory and practice*. Sage, London.

Wiener M (1989) Psychopathology reconsidered. Depression interpreted as psychosocial interactions. *Clinical Psychology Review* 9: 295–321.

Further reading

- Burton M (1998) *Psychotherapy, Counselling and Primary Mental Health Care*. Wiley, Chichester.

- Curtis Jenkins G and Einzig H (1996) Counselling in primary care. In: R Bayne, I Hortgon and J Bimrose (eds) *New Directions in Counselling*. Routledge, London, pp. 97–108.

- East P (1995) *Counselling in Medical Settings*. Open University Press, Buckingham.

- Fairhurst I (ed.) (1999) *Women Writing in the Person Centred Approach*. PCCS Books, Ross-on-Wye.

- Hoyt MF (1995) *Brief Therapy and Managed Care Readings for Contempory Practice*. Jossey Bass, San Francisco, CA.

- Hudson Allez G (1997) *Time Limited Therapy in a General Practice Setting: how to help within six sessions*. Sage, London.

- Keithly J, Bond T and Marsh G (eds) (2002) *Counselling in Primary Care* (2e). Oxford University Press, Oxford.

- Kirschenbaum H and Henderson VL (1990) *The Carl Rogers Reader*. Constable, London.

- Natiello P (2001) *The Person-Centred Approach: a passionate presence*. PCCS Books, Ross-on-Wye.

- Wyatt G (ed.) *Rogers' Therapeutic Conditions: evolution, theory and practice*. 4 vols. PCCS Books, Ross-on-Wye.

Further information

Organisations and journals

Healthcare Counselling and Psychotherapy Journal
British Association for Counselling and Psychotherapy, 1 Regent Place, Rugby
CV21 2PJ.
Tel: 0870 443 5252
Email: hcpj.editorial@bacp.co.uk

Counselling in Primary Care Trust
Tel: 01784 441782
Email: gcurtisjenkins@compuserve.com
http://www.cpct.co.uk
The Counselling in Primary Care Trust has, since its foundation in 1991, promoted, supported and aided the development of counselling in primary healthcare. The charitable Trust has funded research projects, systematic reviews and a number of training initiatives, and has published a quarterly newsletter 'Counselling in Practice', serving the needs of counsellors working in primary healthcare. Counsellit is a unique collection of 2700 references and abstracts collected over the past 17 years by the Counselling in Primary Care Trust. The database is now available as a CD ROM. The collection covers primary healthcare, mental healthcare, psychological therapies including counselling and psychotherapy, supervision, important research trials and other subjects of interest for researchers, students, counsellors and other professional healthcare staff who work in the NHS.

Counsellors and Psychotherapists in Primary Care (CPC)
Queensway House, Queensway, Bognor Regis, West Sussex PO21 1QT.
Tel: 01243 870701
Email: cpc@cpc-online.co.uk
www.cpc-online.co.uk
CPC is the specialist professional membership organisation representing counsellors and psychotherapists working in primary care. It offers a wide range of training courses, publications and consultancy.

British Association for the Person-Centred Approach (BAPCA)
Bm-BAPCA, London WC1N 3XX.
Tel: 01989 770948
Email: info@bapca.org.uk
http://www.bapca.org.uk
National association promoting the person-centred approach. Publishes the journal *Person-centred Practice* and a regular newsletter 'Person-to-Person'.

World Association for Person-Centered and Experiential Psychotherapy and Counselling
Email: secretariat@pce-world.org
http://www.pce-world.org

Association for the Development of the Person-Centered Approach (ADPCA)
Email: adpca-web@signs.portents.com
http://www.adpca.org
An international association, with members in 27 countries, for those interested in the development of client-centred therapy and the person-centred approach.

Person-Centred Therapy Scotland
Tel: 0870 7650871
Email: info@pctscotland.co.uk
www.pctscotland.co.uk
An association of person-centred therapists in Scotland which offers training and networking opportunities to members with the aim of fostering high standards of professional practice.

Index